LIVE LIFE KETO

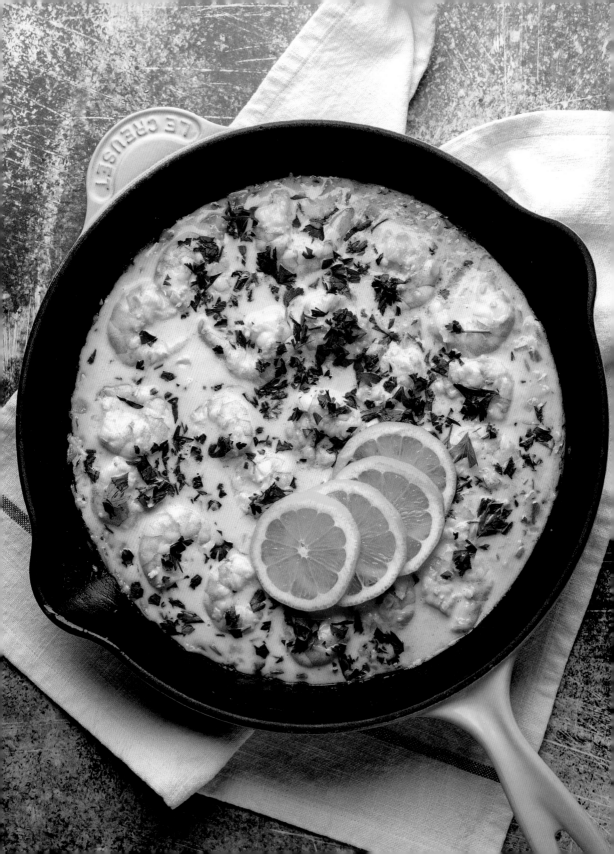

LIVE LIFE KETO

100 Simple Recipes to Live a
Low-Carb Lifestyle and
Lose the Weight for Good

Jennifer Banz

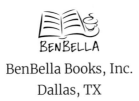
BenBella Books, Inc.
Dallas, TX

BenBella
BenBella Books, Inc.
10440 N. Central Expressway
Suite 800
Dallas, TX 75231
benbellabooks.com
Send feedback to feedback@benbellabooks.com
BenBella is a federally registered trademark.

Printed in the United States of America
10 9 8 7 6 5 4 3 2 1

Library of Congress Control Number: 2022013469
ISBN 9781637741528
eISBN 9781637741535

Editing by Claire Schulz
Copyediting by Michael Fedison
Proofreading by James Fraleigh and Rebecca Maines
Indexing by WordCo
Text design and composition by Aaron Edmiston
Cover design by Sarah Avinger
Cover photography by Jennifer Banz
Printed by Versa Press

To my amazing husband, Matt, and the two most amazing kids in the world, Hayden and Audrey: you are my everything. A lot has changed for the better in our life over the past five years, but none of it would be worth anything without you three by my side.

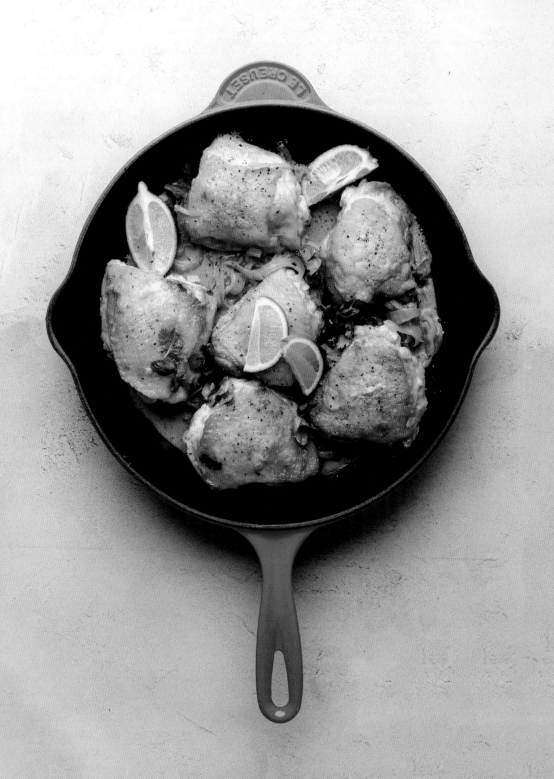

CONTENTS

INTRODUCTION

What if I told you that a diet could help you not only lose weight but have more energy, fewer hunger pangs, and fewer cravings? What if I told you it could help you maintain your goal weight and improve your health for years?

Well, if you're here, you might not be that surprised! By now, you've probably heard of keto. The low-carb keto way of life has increased immensely in popularity over the past few years and there is no question that it works very well. Not only does it help with weight loss, but it also helps improve conditions like diabetes, epilepsy, metabolic syndrome, polycystic ovarian syndrome, migraines—even some cancers. In fact, doctors are increasingly prescribing the keto diet to their patients to help alleviate their symptoms.

The problem? Many people struggle to stick to it. Everyone loves the benefits, but when a diet feels hard to follow, it's too easy to give up. I know—I've been there! That's why I'm writing this cookbook. Not only does it have over one hundred recipes that are easy, fast, and exceptionally delicious, but it also provides a practical resource to help you change your mindset so you can live keto for life.

My Journey to Living Life Keto

I grew up in the South in the '80s and '90s in a typical household. I was a big girl from the beginning, and I thought my weight was out of my control—obesity was in my genes, after all. At the age of four, I was bigger than my friends, and by the time I was in middle school, I was being bullied for my weight. (I'm not saying this so you feel bad for me. Heck, everyone got bullied for something. But if that was you, too, know that I feel your pain!) I liked to eat when I was bored, and I *loved* fast food, chocolate, and ice cream.

I went off and on diets from high school into college, but I could never stick to any one for longer than a week or two. I stayed in the zone of about 100 pounds overweight for most of my early twenties. I played the victim hard—always wondering why I couldn't be skinny like my friends.

I married my husband when I was twenty-eight. He was in the Air Force and got stationed in Germany, so we moved overseas immediately. I had our first child a year later, and my whole outlook on health changed. Now I was taking care of this little person that I loved so much and I didn't want him to suffer with his weight like I did.

Right around this time, the Paleo diet was becoming more popular, and I hoped that eating that way would put my son on a different path than the one I'd walked. He ate avocados and homemade baby food. His first birthday cake was a low-sugar carrot cake that I made from scratch. Secretly, I was hoping switching myself to Paleo would help me lose some

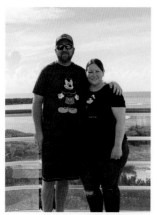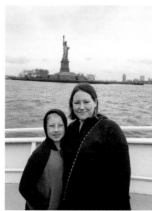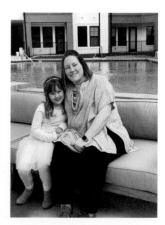

This is me with my husband, my son, and my daughter, right before
I discovered my five fail-stops to living keto for life.

weight, too. I would spend hours scrolling through message boards looking for Paleo weight loss success stories and research. If it wasn't Paleo, I wouldn't be eating it.

I thought the Paleo diet was a magic way to eat that would help my body fat just melt off. I was led to believe that the chemicals in processed food were keeping me fat. Well, unfortunately, I was wrong! You need to eat fewer calories than your body burns to lose weight. Period. I kept slowly gaining weight, eventually hitting 260 pounds.

When my son was two, I decided to have lap-band surgery. This is an inflatable band that is placed around the top portion of the stomach to decrease food consumption. Once again, I thought I had found the magic bullet that was going to help me finally lose weight. I did lose 30 pounds (most was lost during the pre-op liquid diet, and the rest right after surgery). And then I plateaued. My band would be tight in the morning, but by evening time I could eat pretty much whatever I wanted. So, I could still eat enough to keep my weight the same.

With the lap-band, I did have trouble eating certain foods such as breads and pastas. I once again found myself researching how to make the band work for me by reading blogs and message boards. That's how I came across a low-carb approach to eating. My favorite foods were ones filled with sugar and carbs, so I thought if I eliminated those foods, maybe I could lose some weight. And finally, I was on the right track.

My second baby had just turned one, and we had moved back to the States, so over the course of seven months, I went low carb. I always had trouble controlling my intake of sugar- and carb-filled foods—I couldn't eat just a few bites of ice cream and be satisfied. (Let's be honest, it's much easier to eat a big bowl of ice cream than it is to eat an equal-sized bowl of baked chicken!) It was easier if I abstained from those carby foods altogether. My first good, hard try at keto, in 2014 and 2015, was a success. I felt so much better and lost 50 pounds! Still, from time to time I struggled with the temptation to eat sugary and high-carb foods. (We're all human, right?)

In the summer of 2015, our family life changed forever. My husband suffered an injury and had to medically retire from the military. Suddenly, we had to move in with my family across the country while my husband looked for work—and finding a new job took him some months. Needless to say, the stress of life got in the way and I gained all of my weight back.

We finally got back on our feet in early 2016 and my husband found a job as a truck driver. Everything was going okay . . . except he was gone for weeks at a time. This really took a toll on home life. He was always gone, and I was home alone with our two young children. After about six months of this, I decided I would do everything I could to bring him home. I set up a vision board and I tried different ways to make money from home. I tried everything from multi-level marketing to photography. Those were dead ends or took too much time. But I was cooking keto again, so I figured, why not take pictures of my dinner and post it on a food blog? In the fall of 2016, *Low Carb with Jennifer* was born.

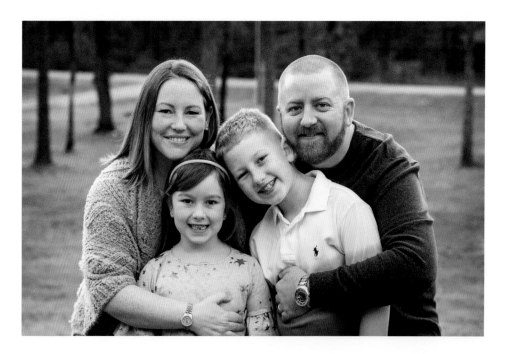

As you've probably picked up by now, I am an avid researcher and dove into find out everything I could about search engine optimization and Pinterest algorithms. So it didn't take long for me to start having success with my little food blog. But it wasn't all algorithms and SEO. Readers came to know me for keto recipes that were actually easy, quick, delicious, and made with ingredients that could be found at any grocery store. My fans started showing up every Thursday at noon for a live keto Q&A session (and answers to many of their FAQs are in the coming chapters!). I made keto realistic so it could work for them.

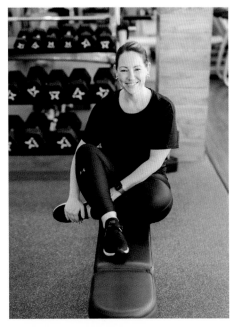

This is me today, living the keto lifestyle!

By April of 2018, I had replaced my husband's income, and two months later, he quit his job to be a stay-at-home dad. Despite our accomplishments, I was still struggling with overeating carbs and sugar, and I stayed right around 100 pounds overweight. I wondered if I was broken in some way. Nothing I did seemed to make a difference for long.

So what changed?

My longtime readers and fans inspired me to go deep and learn about making lasting change. In the spring of 2020, I was introduced to the Life Coach School, and I finally learned how the human brain works. I learned that I was not broken; in fact, my brain was working exactly how it was supposed to. I'll tell you all about this in "Sticking to It" on pages 21–34. I was not a victim of outside circumstances. If I wanted to see success on keto, it would be 90 percent mindset and 10 percent everything else.

Learning about how the brain works, and how we can rewire it for our own advantage, was a game changer for me. With all that I learned and other techniques I will teach you in this book, I have managed to lose 80 pounds, and I know these tools and keto are going to help me keep the weight off for life. And it's how I'm helping my clients lose weight, as well. I now teach what I've learned in my coaching membership, Live Life Keto, and I'm sharing those secrets in this book!

In This Book

This book is for you if you're just getting started with keto, if you've tried it several times but just can't stick to it, or if you're having success with keto and want to make it a lifestyle. I'm here to show you how.

In Part I, we'll cover the basics of going keto and the powerful mindset shifts that help make it possible to stick with the diet. You'll also find a section all about some of my favorite ingredients and some helpful tips for eating keto on the go.

Then, in Part II, you'll find over one hundred recipes that reflect my personal philosophy on cooking: everything has got to be simple, fast, and exceptionally delicious. And no obscure ingredients or things you'll only use once and then leave sitting around gathering dust in your pantry. I hope you'll find many new favorite dishes that you'll enjoy again and again. But I really hope you'll find something else . . .

Believe in Your Own Badassery

If you take anything away from this book, I want it to be the belief in yourself.

You can do this. You can reach your goal weight. If you don't believe it, your road will be much longer and harder. But guess what? You can decide right now that you believe in yourself. It really is just as easy as a simple thought! *I believe in myself. I believe that I can reach my goal weight.* Look in the mirror and say it or write it in a journal every single day and eventually you will truly believe it as truth.

This is true for all of us! We have to call ourselves out on our own BS and change our mentality so we can live the lives we've always wanted. We can do it any time we want. We are in control of our weight, our bank account, our happiness, and our destiny. I know it sounds cliché, but when you believe it, you can achieve it.

It's not magic. When we believe something, like *I know I will definitely reach my goal weight*, we start to take steps to *make* it true. (It really wouldn't make sense to believe you can reach your goal weight, but then take completely opposite actions—like sitting on the couch all day while eating candy bars.) Look into the future and see the future self of your dreams. How does she look, act, eat, dress, exercise, and respond to stress? You've got to look in the mirror and believe in yourself. You've got to start being your future self *right now.*

Now that you know this about yourself—you are in control of your own thoughts, feelings, actions, and results and you are not a victim of outside circumstances—what are you going to do about it? It's time to see what you are capable of. Take what you learn in this book and apply it to anything you want in your life. What do you think you can do after you conquer this weight loss hurdle? Make a million dollars? Travel the world? Quit your draining job? You are UNSTOPPABLE and you are in control.

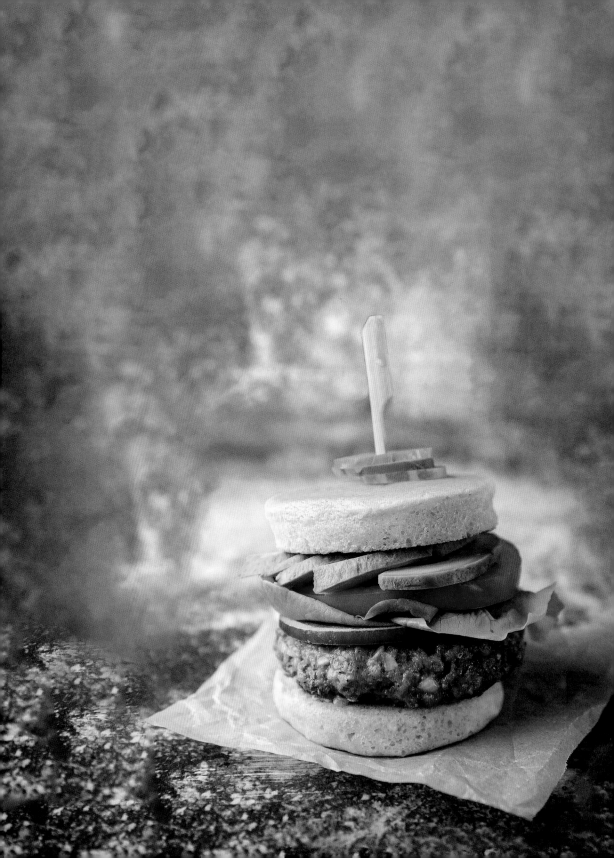

Part I:

LIVING LIFE KETO

GETTING STARTED

The Basics of Keto

What is all this ruckus about keto? It seemed like a fad diet at first, but it's just not going away, is it? For this I am thankful because without keto, I would not be where I am today. I wouldn't have my blog, *Low Carb with Jennifer*; I would not have lost over 80 pounds; and I would not have written this book!

So what exactly is keto and why is it better for weight loss than all the other fads out there? I get this question a lot and I never get tired of answering it. I just want to shout all about keto from the rooftops. Not only is it wonderfully effective for weight loss, but it has helped so many people to prevent or manage health issues such as insulin resistance, type 2 diabetes, high blood pressure, fatty liver, polycystic ovarian syndrome (PCOS), migraines, arthritis, and many others. It's a life-changer.

If you've been eating keto for a while, you may want to skip this chapter and get right into "Sticking to It" on page 21, where you'll find the mindset tips to help you keep going. If that's you, go for it! If you are just getting started, or you'd like some refreshers, this chapter lays out the basics—Keto 101, if you will—so you can set yourself up for success.

What Is Keto?

Keto is the short name for a ketogenic diet, or a way of eating that switches the body into ketosis. To put it in simplest terms, ketosis is a process where your body burns fat for energy instead of carbohydrates. Getting a little more technical, it is a natural metabolic state in which your liver is producing ketones instead of glucose for fuel. Don't yawn and close the book just yet—I promise I will not get into too much scientific jargon, but this is important to understand! All food is composed of three macronutrients (macros): carbohydrates, protein, and fat. When we eat carbohydrates, our bodies break it down into glucose—most of our cells' preferred form of fuel. The pancreas then releases the hormone insulin, which helps to transport that glucose all throughout the body. This is a normal process, but when we get too much insulin, it can lead to excess body fat, cause dramatic rises and drops in energy, and put us at risk of health conditions like insulin resistance, type 2 diabetes, heart disease, and more.

When we're fasting or restricting our carb intake, the body doesn't get that glucose for fuel. Our insulin levels stay low, and the liver starts breaking down fats into "ketone bodies" (or "ketones") that it can use for energy instead. Being in ketosis helps you lose weight because you're burning fat for energy. And over the long term, a keto diet can naturally lower your appetite, meaning you'll take in fewer calories.

What's more, eating foods that are low in carbs and sugar keeps our insulin low. When our insulin is low, we are not on the blood sugar roller coaster and we have constant sustained energy (that means no 2 PM sugar crashes).

So we know we want our liver producing ketones for fuel because that means our body is burning fat more than glucose (sugar) and our insulin is low. How do we start this process and become a fat-burning machine instead of a sugar burner?

Keto is as easy as three simple steps focused on those macros. We need to limit carbohydrates, prioritize protein, and fill with fat.

Limit Carbohydrates

Limiting carbs is really the most important piece to this puzzle. We have to limit carbohydrates in order to reach a state of ketosis. So what does that mean? I'm glad you asked!

To start ketosis, you need to limit your intake of carbohydrates to 20–50 grams per day. (The exact number varies between individuals. Generally, it's safe to stick to around 20–30 grams of net carbs per day to stay in ketosis; for more on net carbs, see the box on the next page.) In contrast, someone following a standard American diet is averaging 260 grams of carbohydrates per day.

What foods are high in carbohydrates? These are typically any sugary or starchy foods like breads, grains, pasta, beans, rice, and fruits and vegetables such as potatoes, apples, and bananas. The best way to figure out if a food is keto-friendly is to look at the food label (check the carbohydrates per serving) or, if there's no label, do a quick search online. You want to select foods that are lowest in carbohydrates. Most of your carbs should come from non-starchy vegetables like leafy greens, squash, asparagus, broccoli, Brussels sprouts, cauliflower, and small servings of berries.

Net Carbs

If you've started following any low-carb diet advice, you've probably heard the term "net carbs" thrown around a lot. It's true that it's more important to look at net carbs than total carbs when you're calculating your intake. So what are they? Net carbs are the carbohydrates in food that you can actually digest and process for fuel—the ones that increase blood sugar. Fiber and sugar alcohols (like erythritol and xylitol) are included in a food's total carb count, but our bodies don't digest them—they simply pass through us. To calculate net carbs, simply take the total carbs in a food (in grams) and subtract the fiber and sugar alcohols.

For example, Lakanto Monkfruit Sweetener's nutrition label says it has 8 grams of carbohydrates and 8 grams of sugar alcohols. Therefore, this product has zero net carbs (8 carbs – 8 sugar alcohols = 0 net carbs).

One medium banana has 27 grams of carbohydrates and 3 grams of fiber. Therefore it has 24 net carbs (27 grams of carbs – 3 grams of fiber = 24 net carbs).

I recommend sticking to around 20–30 grams of net carbs per day if you want to maintain ketosis.

Prioritize Protein

Next up is protein, which is often overlooked in a ketogenic diet. Protein is important because it helps keep you satisfied, your body needs it to repair and build tissue and regulate your thyroid hormones, and it can act as an energy source if needed. I recommend at least 100 grams of protein per day. No matter what diet you choose, you should always prioritize protein.

What keto-friendly foods are a great protein source? That would be any meat, poultry, or seafood, eggs, and low-sugar protein powders.

Fill with Fat

Fat is our final macronutrient but it's definitely not the least important. Our bodies require fat for many functions including hormone production and keeping our gallbladder healthy. (Are you wondering why so many people, especially women, are having to have their gallbladders removed? It's because they do not eat enough fat! When you restrict fat, your liver doesn't need to produce bile to digest the fat in the intestines. So the bile sits in the gallbladder, turns into thick sludge, and eventually forms stones. Yikes!) Fat helps us to absorb certain vitamins, protect our organs, and keep us warm. And fat helps us to feel full and satisfied when we eat, which is particularly important when we change our diet. Especially on keto, you may find yourself craving sugary or starchy foods, and fat can help to counteract that.

Quality fats are a crucial component of a healthy diet, but you may have heard otherwise from someone pushing a low-fat regimen. Saturated fat, which is fat from animals, has been villainized for far too long as a major driver of heart disease. In fact, a meta-analysis of over 72 published studies concluded that saturated fats had no effect on heart health and it was trans fats (the ones found in baked goods, fried foods, and margarine) that were the culprits all along. Keep in mind that fat is very calorie dense so we should satisfy our hunger with fat but not go overboard. If you hear of someone who tried the keto diet but didn't lose weight, they were probably overeating fat. Your target fat intake for a day will depend on your personal daily calorie goal (see page 16).

What are good fat sources for keto? Choose sources of fat that naturally occur with protein, like a fatty steak or fatty fish like salmon. Also prioritize full-fat dairy and butter, avocados, coconut oil, olive oil, nuts, nut butters, and seeds.

A Day in the Keto Life

Here is how a typical day looks for me following a ketogenic diet:

Breakfast: Coffee with half-and-half and sugar-free sweetener, a serving of Ham and Swiss Breakfast Casserole (page 53).

Lunch: Another cup of coffee with half-and-half and sugar-free sweetener, a keto-friendly soup like my Steak and Fauxtato Soup (page 87), and a cup of strawberries.

Dinner: My Favorite Salmon Salad Meal Prep (page 116).

This day provides me with approximately 1,700 calories, 29 grams of total carbohydrates, 11 grams of fiber, 100 grams of protein, and 135 grams of fat.

How Much Do I Eat?

Isn't that the million-dollar question? Like I said in the introduction, you must eat in a calorie deficit to lose weight, plain and simple. But the exact number depends on your sex, age, height, how active you are, and how much you currently weigh. So it's important to find out what will work for *you*. My favorite calorie calculator can be found online at www.calculator .net/calorie-calculator.html. When you input your information accurately,

Keto-Friendly Food Choices

Do a search online for calorie and carb counts for specific foods. This is just to get you started, not an exhaustive list!

Protein	Meats (beef, pork, lamb, game) Poultry (chicken, turkey)	Eggs Fish and seafood Low-carb protein powder
Dairy	Butter Cream cheese Cheeses	Greek yogurt (unsweetened) Heavy cream and half-and-half
Fats and oils	Avocado oil Olive oil Butter	Beef tallow Duck fat Nut butters
Non-starchy vegetables and low-sugar fruits	Artichoke hearts Asparagus Avocados Berries (low-sugar, in small portions) Broccoli Brussels sprouts Cauliflower Celery Cucumber Herbs and spices	Leafy greens Lemons Limes Mushrooms Olives Onions Peppers (bell peppers, jalapenos) Radishes Watermelon
Nuts and seeds	Almonds Almond flour Chia seeds	Poppy seeds Sesame seeds
Condiments and sweeteners	Mayonnaise Sour cream	Sugar-free sweeteners (erythritol, monkfruit, xylitol)

it will give you calorie counts to maintain your weight, lose 0.5 pounds a week, 1 pound a week, or 2 pounds a week.

You may notice how few calories the calculator will indicate if you want to lose 2 pounds a week. Why has 2 pounds a week been deemed the expectation? If you were to ask anyone how much weight they expect to lose per week, chances are, they would say 2 pounds. We always want the weight loss to happen faster. But for a lot of us, faster is unsustainable because of the way our brain works. (More on this in the next chapter.) It is almost impossible to lose that much weight per week sustainably—expecting to follow that over time is setting yourself up for failure. A much more realistic goal is 1 pound per week. So set that number as your target.

Keeping Track

Some people keep track of their macros and calories on paper and some keep track with an app on their phone. I am an advocate for the phone and I love keeping track of my food with the My Fitness Pal app, which is free and very easy to use. You can search for a food or you can scan a packaged food's barcode and it will calculate everything for you. This isn't the only food tracking app by any means, so feel free to try a few and pick your favorite.

You may have tried to limit your calorie intake before and found it a challenge. Keto is very helpful at regulating our hunger hormones so we do not usually overeat. A lot of people find weight loss success just by reducing their carbs to the recommended 20–30 net carbs per day. But what about those of us who have a habit of eating when we're not even hungry? We have to learn to eat when we are hungry and stop when we are satisfied.

For a lot of people this is very tough to learn. That's why I recommend tracking your food intake anytime you find that you stop losing weight for more than three weeks. You will already be tracking your carbohydrates to maintain a state of ketosis, so you might as well track your calories while you are at it!

Counting calories has gotten a bad rap recently, but there is nothing wrong with tracking your intake. I equate it to tracking your finances. If you wanted to save money, you would make a budget and monitor your spending to make sure you were staying on target.

> **Keto Basics at a Glance**
> If you aim to lose weight, you must eat fewer calories than needed to maintain your body weight. Find your daily target using an online calculator. Then, aim for:
> - 20-30 grams net carbs
> - 100 grams of protein
> - Healthy fats in moderation

What About the "Keto Flu"?

I'm sure you've heard of the keto flu, and it might actually be deterring you from trying keto. It really isn't that big of a deal, and it is easy to get over with a few simple steps. But let's back up a minute and talk about why it happens. Keto flu happens because we are switching from burning carbohydrates to burning fat. Our body is looking for those carbs, but they are being depleted. We can feel run-down and low on energy for about a week and then it's usually back to normal, or better than normal! We are also expelling a lot of electrolytes (sodium and magnesium) with the water weight "whoosh" that usually comes with switching to keto.

Some things you can do to make life a little easier during this transition are to make sure you are getting enough rest, staying hydrated, and getting enough salt in your diet. You can also combat some of the symptoms with a magnesium supplement, but this is something I have rarely had to do.

What About Keto Convenience Foods?

If you go to any keto support group online, you may have a run-in with the "keto police." These are the people who are quick to judge our personal choices and will quickly tell you a food you enjoy isn't keto-friendly. This type of judgment from others is very loud, but we do not have to listen to it. We are free to form our own opinions and eat keto the way that works for us.

In my opinion, the food you eat is a personal choice, and if you eat 30 grams net carbs or less, congratulations! You are eating keto! I never stress about the sugar in my bacon, the sucralose in my sugar-free BBQ sauce, or the milk in my plain Greek yogurt. If it fits in my macros for the day, it's keto for me. If you want to eat the keto bread from Costco, please do. If you want a quesadilla made with a low-carb tortilla, be my guest. If you enjoy the occasional diet soda, no judgment here—I do, too! Don't let anyone tell you that you are doing keto wrong.

There are a lot of keto convenience foods out there and they are very helpful for people like me and you to help us stay on track. Without these foods, we might just go back to eating how we were eating before keto, and that's definitely not what we want. I consider these convenience foods the halfway point to optimal eating. Optimal eating or "clean keto" would be a life totally based on whole foods, without convenience foods that contain questionable ingredients, gluten, or nonnatural sweeteners—not a very realistic goal, if you ask me. As long as you're aware that some keto convenience foods might tempt you to overeat fat or calories (see the next chapter for more), and you can keep hitting your goals, I consider this "halfway" eating much better than the alternative.

Most of us, including myself, will probably never make it to 100 percent optimal eating and there is absolutely nothing wrong with that. What good is striving for perfection when it is impossible to stick to?

Speaking of sticking to it—now that you've mastered the basics of keto, we'll talk about some common challenges that people have with staying keto long term.

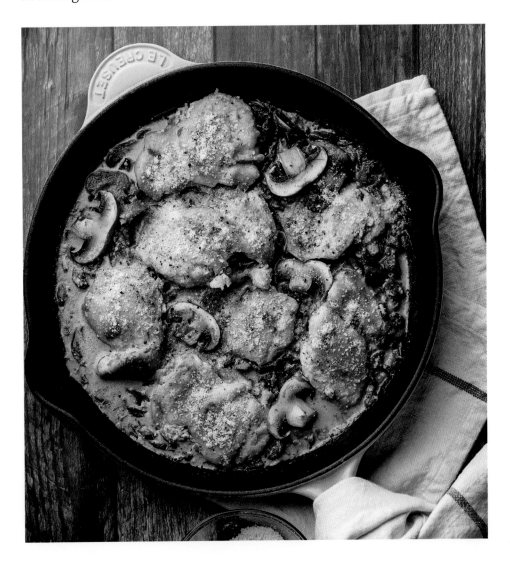

STICKING TO IT

The 5 Fail-Stops to Stay on Course

Many times, my clients and readers will ask, "Why is keto so hard to stick to?" I understand where they are coming from. But let's be clear—it's not just keto that is hard to stick to. Absolutely every diet that is out there to help with weight loss can be hard. In fact, diet compliance is pretty low across the board, with only 25 percent of participants sticking with *any* diet long term.

Why is that? Why only 25 percent compliance? Well, there are a few reasons. One is that foods these days, particularly the unhealthier ones, are made to make us crave them. Another is pressure from others to "eat normal" and not rock the boat. And the toughest is that our own thoughts and mindset can put hurdles in our way. This chapter is all about how you can stick to your keto plan and enjoy life—despite all the hyper-palatable foods, pressure from others, and your own brain trying to knock you off course. You've gotten off to a great start with your keto basics, and now you're moving on to the advanced level. Remember, you got this! I believe in you.

Breaking the Spell of Craveable Foods

Look around you. We are bombarded with images and messages pushing food. They are all over the TV, on almost every street corner, and now just a swipe on the phone away via online food delivery. Most often, these ads and images show us foods that are processed and are made with a mix of fat, salt, carbohydrates, and sugar—what health experts call hyper-palatable foods, which are designed to "light up" our reward center in our lower brain. I also call them craveable foods because our lower brain remembers how delicious they were, and how good it felt to eat them, so the brain craves more and more. We never really crave a bowl of plain pasta. It alone isn't hyper-palatable. But when we add the sauce and cheese? We crave it. The same goes for a plain pizza crust. That really doesn't sound very appealing, does it? Now add all the toppings and we have our hyper-palatable, craveable food. Food companies know this, and they have formulas to develop the food so it is so good we can't help but keep eating. Recognizing this, we can make a conscious choice to stop or to choose a healthier option.

Keep in mind, this doesn't apply to just conventional junk food or fast food. Even keto processed foods like those keto protein bars, cookies, shakes, and chips are more than likely made hyper-palatable, too. The foods' manufacturers want their product to be really delicious so we keep buying them and their companies stay in business.

Now, that's not to say that keto convenience foods can have no place in your life. As I mentioned in the last chapter, these "halfway" options can help make it easier for you to stick with keto. Perfection isn't the goal. Long-term success is. And if eating these foods (in moderation!) helps you stick to your new normal, then by all means, enjoy them! Just be sure they aren't tempting you to overeat and miss your macronutrient and calorie targets.

Embracing Your New Normal

"But, Jennifer, I just want to eat normal!" This is something I get a lot. Many people think with a diet mentality when they decide to try to lose weight. They think, *I'm going to eat this way temporarily, and then go back to eating normal after I reach my goal weight.* But I want you to think about what is *really* normal eating, and what society tells us is normal.

When early humans' large brains developed, their diet—our human diet—involved lots of meat and fat. We had animals we hunted for, plants we could forage, and some seasonal fruit and honeycomb. We ate the whole animal, nose to tail. When food was available, we likely ate only a couple of times a day and fasted a lot, meaning our insulin levels lowered between meals, and so our bodies would continue to burn fat. This was truly normal eating for humans for hundreds of thousands of years, before the advent of agriculture brought us plentiful cultivated wheat, and the Industrial Revolution eventually paved the way for mass-produced processed foods. At some point, advice shifted from eating fewer, bigger meals to eating many small meals a day to "keep your metabolism going."

"Normal" in our society today is eating six or more times a day, three large meals, snacks, and dessert, meaning our insulin is always elevated and our bodies are not efficient at burning fat. It's "normal" to have alcohol every day. It's "normal" to always eat cake and ice cream at parties, pile our plates with sweets during the holidays, and down nachos, pizza, and beer while watching football. We have normalized overeating so much so that when we are trying to eat less, everyone thinks something is wrong with us!

So when we try to stick with a diet, we just want to go back to eating the way we were used to because we are trying to go with the flow of society and the food is just plain delicious. Humans do not like to be different or seen as different from their peers. It creates a lot of tension internally. Our brains are wired to be socially accepted. (We'll get to some ways to shift your mindset later in this chapter to help with this!)

What I want you to do is redefine normal eating for yourself. You can't look outside of yourself to define what's normal because that "normal" eating has created a society where more than two-thirds of adults are over-weight and millions of us struggle with chronic diseases and conditions including insulin resistance, type 2 diabetes, high blood pressure, fatty liver disease, and PCOS. No matter what way of eating we choose to lose weight and keep it off, we have to let some of this food go most of the time. The rich pasta dishes, bread baskets, chips and salsa, ice cream sundaes, giant bagels with cream cheese, 300-calorie cups of coffee—we can't eat this stuff every day and expect to lose weight or maintain a healthy weight. *Your* new normal has to be the way you eat that can consistently give you the healthy body and life that you want—and then you eat that way for the rest of your life.

I hate when people tell me they could never eat keto because then they could never have "fun" food again, like "real" cake or ice cream or cookies. That really couldn't be further from the truth! You have to enjoy the process because if you think this way of eating is hard, boring, restrictive, or not fun, unfortunately, you will quit. Living your life keto doesn't mean never having your favorite bakery treat or your grandma's brownies again. I still have "real" cake and ice cream and cookies! The difference is that I used to eat that stuff almost daily. Now, I choose to limit it to once a week and I plan it in advance (more on this later). So I'm not saying you can never have those foods again. I'm saying that eating those foods is not your "normal" anymore. When you do indulge in them, you enjoy the treat without guilt and then it's right back to your normal keto routine. You can also make room in your repertoire for more delicious *and* keto-friendly desserts and snacks, like my favorite yogurt parfait on page 237.

The 5 Fail-Stops to Stick to Your New Normal

We know that keto is a great plan for weight loss and eating this way has many benefits for health. The real question is, how do we stick with keto for life in a world filled with hyper-palatable foods that are pushed on us and pressure from others to fit in?

These five fail-stops have been my secret to sticking with keto and losing weight. Without these fail-stops, there is no doubt in my mind I would be laid up on the couch with a bowl of chips instead of writing this book. I would not have been able to make keto my lifestyle.

Having these fail-stops in place is key to sticking with any weight loss plan. We all know what it takes to lose weight—committing to a diet that works and sticking to it—but we have many obstacles to navigate, including in our own mindset. It's how we handle these obstacles that determines our success.

The five fail-stops are:

1. Determine your "why"
2. Plan ahead
3. Get uncomfortable
4. Stop the self-judgment
5. Manage overwhelm

In the rest of this chapter, we'll look at each in more detail.

Fail-Stop 1: Determine Your "Why"

It's such a cliché to ask, but—why do you want to do this? Most people would say they want to lose weight, become a size 6, or go off their medications, and stop at that. But are any of those goals truly compelling? They're not, and that's why we end up quitting most of the time. So why do you want to be a size 6? Why do you want to get off of your medications? Why do you want to look good in a bikini? We have to answer those questions and go even deeper.

You want to lose weight. Why?

So you will live a long life pain free. But why is that important?

Is it so you can play on the floor with your kids or grandkids? Or how about watching your grandkids grow up? Maybe you want to be able to fly on an airplane without the need for a seat belt extender or feel comfortable riding all of the amusement park rides.

We tend to forget that as life progresses, we do not stay the same. We go down a path of aging, and being in an unhealthy state further complicates that fact.

So, in one, five, or ten years, your health could take a turn for the worse, or it could take a turn for the better depending on what you choose *right now.*

Imagine yourself ten years from now without having taken any action toward better health.

How would you feel physically? Would you have gained more weight? How much? Would any physical ailment be worse?

How would you feel mentally?

How would your overall health be? What specific concerns do you have for your health?

How would you look?

Now, imagine yourself ten years from now after you *have* taken actions to improve your health.

How would you feel physically? What physical activities could you do?

How would you feel mentally?

How much better would your health be? Could you potentially be off of medications?

How would you look? Could you shop at different stores?

The answers to these questions are fuel to my fire and what keep me going. My goal isn't to be a size 6. I couldn't care less what size I am! My "why" is to be able to walk without a walker when I am 90. My "why" is to be strong and healthy for my kids and future grandkids.

Now don't answer these questions and completely forget about them. Write your "why" down on note cards and read them every day. Read them when you wake up and before you go to bed. Read them when you want to eat something that's not on your plan or when you don't want to exercise. These are the fuel to your fire.

Fail-Stop 2: Plan Ahead

Planning is essential when we want to accomplish any goal. So the second sharpest tool in my tool shed, behind finding my why, is to make a plan and stick to it. This includes weekly food prepping, a daily food plan, and an exercise plan. Yes, I write down exactly what I am going to eat and how I am going to exercise every morning (or the day before), and then I follow that plan. If you're not already planning your meals and workouts, I recommend you do it, too.

How does this help us? It all comes down to how our brains work. When we plan ahead, we are using our prefrontal cortex, or our planning brain—the part that's responsible for problem solving, reasoning, and impulse control. This is the part of the brain that knows exactly what we need to do to get the job done. This is the part that probably bought this book! The planning brain has a counterpart, though: the primal brain (also known as the lower brain or sometimes the lizard brain). This is the part of the brain that is more instinctive and reactive, and it's the part that can trip us up on the path to achieving our goals.

We make hundreds of decisions per day. As the day wears on, we get tired having to think everything through—a state psychologists refer to as decision fatigue—and the reactive primal brain can start to take the reins. That's why at the end of a busy day, we would much rather make the easy choice of takeout pizza instead of the better choice of steak and broccoli.

It is time to take the reins back by simply making a plan. Our prefrontal cortex wants the best for us, and by using it to plan ahead, we're overriding the primal brain's impulses. It really is that simple!

I like to plan out my meals either the night before or the morning of my day. I pull out my journal or my phone app, and I go ahead and decide ahead of time what I am going to eat for the day. If I have food prepped and ready to go in the refrigerator, then this step is pretty easy. I'll write down what I am going to eat for breakfast, lunch, and dinner. You might like to plan a day ahead or you might like to plan out your whole week every Sunday night. Do whatever makes life easiest for you—if a week at a time feels overwhelming, well, you don't have to. Day to day has been great for me (with the exception of planning my "exception" foods—more on that in a minute).

Meal prepping is another big part of the planning fail-stop. Prepping food might be the last thing you want to do on a Sunday afternoon. But I can assure you that doing this one thing consistently has kept me on track more than anything. Knowing I already have prepped food in the refrigerator when I get home from a busy day is the best feeling. The trick is to find a prepping routine you enjoy. I love grilling, so every Sunday you will find me grilling a whole bunch of chicken, steak, and burgers for my family for the week. I look forward to prepping food now because I found a way to enjoy it. Seeing a big batch of nourishing protein in my refrigerator that I know can feed my whole family all week is very rewarding!

Planning ahead also includes planning things that wouldn't be considered keto, and this is where longer-term planning comes in handy. Let's say you have a birthday party to attend where you know there will be cake. It is perfectly acceptable (as far as I am concerned) to plan in advance to have a piece of that cake. By choosing to have the cake and enjoy it, you are honoring your plan and avoiding the alternative—*not* planning for the cake, eating it anyway, and then feeling guilty. I call these exceptions, not cheats, because they are an exception to our normal food but there's nothing wrong with them, from time to time, as part of your long-term keto lifestyle. When you are trying to lose weight, I would limit these exceptions to once a week.

When you sit down to plan, some drama can come up in your brain. You may start to think something like: *But, Jennifer, what if I have a last-minute dinner date with a friend? What if my husband eats my planned lunch? What if I get hurt and can't go for a run that day?* Your primal brain may even try to convince you to not make the plan at all because of the thought *You're not going to stick to it anyway, so why even try?*

Guess what? Those questions come straight from your reactive primal brain. It thinks making a plan is the worst idea in the world. By planning, you are taking away all of his pleasure! (Yes, I talk about my primal brain like he has a personality. Because he does! He is like a little inner monster that just wants to lie on the couch and watch Netflix while eating pizza. By making a plan and then sticking to it, we are overriding that little monster and getting closer to our goals.)

We want to make it really complicated. But my answer to all of those *what-if* questions is really simple: "Do the best you can."

If you planned a salad with chicken for lunch but your friend called and wants to go out to dinner, you have a choice to make. You can tell them you can't go. You can go and eat whatever you want and not honor your plan. Or you can go and do the best you can. I always like the latter choice. In any situation, we always have that available to us. Almost all restaurants have meat and vegetables (check out "Keto on the Go" on pages 40–42 for more ideas). Do the best you can.

Fail-Stop 3: Get Uncomfortable

Losing weight is not a walk in the park (though taking one can definitely help). There is no magic pill or trick to losing weight—not even keto!—so stop trying to find it. It's not there. You still have to eat in a calorie deficit to lose weight. That means we have to get comfortable with being uncomfortable. It's not going to be easy, but it is definitely going to be worth it.

The food we have now is some of the tastiest, most hyper-palatable food we have ever had and it's only getting better!

We are also finding easier and easier ways to do everyday things, like using grocery delivery for our weekly grocery shopping. Heck, you can even buy a car online without leaving your house! These are great conveniences. But as they make our lives easier, we get more and more used to them—so the second we try something that feels difficult, we want to give up. Let's get uncomfortable.

Being willing to get uncomfortable is the ticket to your dreams. I get asked all the time: How do I deal with cravings? I get uncomfortable. I have a craving and I let it be there because I know cravings pass. How do I stay motivated to work out? I get uncomfortable and I do what I said I was going to do. If my plan says lift weights for 30 minutes, I lift weights for 30 minutes, even when I don't want to.

Do you think I have more motivation than you? I definitely do not! Some days I don't want to do any of my workouts or eat any of my planned food. But I get uncomfortable and do it anyway because I know that is the ticket to achieving my dreams and going after my "why." Even Olympic athletes don't always want to get up and do their workouts, but they know it's what they need to do if they want to reach their goals, so they do it anyway.

I always wanted to be one of those people who just *wanted* to eat healthy whole foods and exercise every day, and I couldn't figure out what was wrong with me. Why did I keep giving in to hyper-palatable foods like ice cream and cookies? Why couldn't I stay consistent with my exercise? What I didn't realize was that we can be anything we want to be, as long as we believe that that's who we are. When I started believing I was that person, when I started being disciplined with my food and workouts, and when I stopped waiting on motivation and just got uncomfortable, everything changed.

If you are willing to be uncomfortable, you get to see what you are capable of. This means not eating that snack when it's not on your plan for the day, pushing yourself in a workout, or saying no to a dear friend when they want to go shopping and you're trying to save money.

On that note: we also need to be willing to let others be uncomfortable. How often do you give in to the appetizers at a party because you are afraid someone will think you are strange for not eating? Or give in to ordering a slice of pie after dinner with a friend because they do not want to have dessert alone? We are letting them be comfortable at our own expense. We are choosing their pleasure over our own goals. Never be afraid to say no, no matter how uncomfortable everyone else gets. I hope you always choose your own goals over someone else's comfort.

Fail-Stop 4: Stop the Self-Judgment

I have tried a lot of diets all throughout my life and every time I failed, I would be flooded with self-judgment. Why couldn't I just stick to this diet? Why do I eat so much? Why can't I be like one of those fitness models on Instagram?

Every time we ask ourselves why we can't do something, or we add "should" or "shouldn't" into the sentence, we are judging. We could be judging ourselves or someone else.

The problem with "shoulding" all over yourself (or someone else) is that it doesn't serve you (or them). If you are like me, there are times when you have thought, *You should have stuck to that diet longer. You shouldn't have eaten that cake. You should have gone to the gym yesterday.* Stop it right this minute! We are judging ourselves for something that we did or didn't do in the past—something that we now have no control over and cannot change. Seriously, I have known people who judge themselves so hard that they get stuck on the past and cannot move forward.

A friend of mine once lost almost 100 pounds. Then life and old habits got in the way, and she gained nearly all of the weight back. And that was all she could think about: how she *shouldn't* have gained her weight back and she *should* have stuck to her plan. It preoccupied her mind so much that she couldn't actually focus on getting back on track!

What if, instead of judging ourselves, we just acknowledged it happened and moved on? This one mindset shift will keep you from getting too far gone if you start to gain some weight back or aren't seeing the results you want. This fail-stop has kept me from wallowing in self-pity and self-judgment anytime I start to go off track. I still have moments when I fall off track and eat things I wished I hadn't. Sometimes I might go off track for weeks at a time! But two things keep me coming back to keto. One, I know it works and I am confident it is how humans are supposed to eat. And two, I never judge myself for what I have done in the past. This clears my head so I can focus on the future.

I always remember that hyper-palatable foods are surrounding us at virtually every corner. It's no wonder we fall off track every now and then. Honestly, it happens to most people—the ones who never eat off plan are unicorns. Remembering this brings me so much comfort and I hope it does for you, too. You are not broken for eating something off keto. Everything is working just as expected. You are human.

Fail-Stop 5: Manage Overwhelm

If I told you ketosis was only possible if you never ate sugar again for the rest of your life, would you do it? If I said that to lose weight you have to stop eating all of your favorite foods, would you?

My guess is probably not. These types of expectations make us overwhelmed so we quit before we even get started. These are the types of expectations we try to put on ourselves—this diet perfectionism—but striving for 100 percent rarely works and usually leads to bingeing on sugar or quitting.

Our brains are going to give us so many excuses to not get started because of feeling overwhelmed with all that you think you need to do, how perfect you have to be, and how long it's going to take. But eating keto is really simple, and the best advice I can give is to just take it one step at a time.

So often we start thinking about things like, *How am I going to continue doing this one year from now or five years from now?* Then here come the feelings of overwhelm, flooding through the body. When those thoughts or questions pop up into my brain, I quickly shut it down with my favorite mantra: *I can do this today.*

When we let overwhelming thoughts get the best of us, we do things we regret. The thoughts usually come when we see something we really crave—like a giant piece of chocolate cake. The thought of wanting it seems so overwhelming, it is hard to say no in the moment. But just like I said in the planning fail-stop, you can have your cake! Just plan for it. I remind myself, "I can do this today," and I add the cake to my plan as an exception for some day in the future. (Most times you will find that the cravings go away and you don't even want to eat the cake the next day.)

Other overwhelming thoughts, like *I need to lose weight fast*, cause us to try to lose weight in an unsustainable way. We cut our food intake way too low, and then our primal brain takes over once again: it thinks it's starving and goes into a cycle of bingeing and restricting. Humans evolved essentially binge eating. Early humans never had an abundance of food waiting for them in a pantry or refrigerator. When we had food available, we ate as much as we could because we didn't know when our next meal would be. Not much has changed with our brains now. We still have the urge to eat and have not evolved enough to catch up with modern conveniences. So make sure you are not restricting too much. Too much hunger can lead to binge eating. Like I said before, slow weight loss should be the norm. Slow and steady wins the race.

And that's that—the five fail-stops to help you stay on track and see real, lasting results. Losing weight is nothing more than a mental game. Managing your mind is the ticket to living the life of your dreams!

Another part of setting yourself up for success is making sure you have the ingredients you need in your kitchen. Turn to the next chapter to learn more.

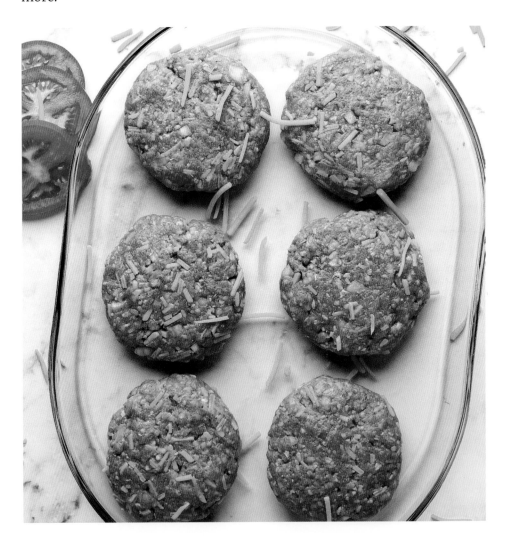

STOCKING YOUR KETO KITCHEN

Must-Have Ingredients and Equipment

First, let's cover the basics! When you make a switch to keto, prioritize meat, non-starchy vegetables, low-sugar fruits like berries, nuts and seeds, no-sugar-added dairy products, and eggs. We all have different tastes, so I don't want to give you an exhaustive (and exhausting!) list of all the ingredients out there. You can do a quick Google search to find out how much of those macros—protein, fat, and carbohydrates—a food contains. For prepackaged foods, when in doubt, always look at the food label for the carb count.

In my keto recipes, I often use six superpowered ingredients that are great to keep stocked in your pantry or refrigerator. You may be unfamiliar with a few of them, but almost all of the other ingredients I use are common ingredients that you can find in just about any grocery store! What's more, because keto has increased in popularity over the years, it is much easier to find keto-friendly foods, even the more unusual ones, wherever you go. Most grocery stores now carry versions of the following ingredients and if not, you can always order them online.

Before we jump in, please be assured you do *not* need to run out and spend hundreds of dollars tomorrow filling your kitchen with keto-friendly foods. I always build up slowly. Pick a few new recipes per week, and just buy the ingredients required along with some extra protein and vegetables to fill in the gaps. Over time, you'll build up a well-stocked keto kitchen ready to take on any recipe!

My Go-To Ingredients

Almond Flour: This is essentially ground almonds and my preferred flour for keto baked goods—I love using almond flour to make keto muffins, breads, cakes, and cookies, and as a replacement for breadcrumbs. Not only is it keto-friendly, it is gluten-free, so it is a great substitute for those who are allergic to gluten or have celiac disease. These days, almond flour is available in most grocery stores, but if you are having trouble finding it, you can grind up whole almonds into a fine powder using a spice grinder.

Avocado Oil: I use avocado oil almost exclusively as my cooking oil of choice because it has a higher smoke point than cooking fats such as olive oil or butter. The smoke point is the temperature at which the oil begins to smoke and oxidize. You can find avocado oil almost anywhere now as it has increased in popularity over the years.

Cauliflower Rice: This is simply cauliflower that has been pulsed in a food processor until it resembles rice. Now you can find it already made in the frozen section of most grocery stores. Use it anytime you need a rice fix! You may also be surprised to see it in my Hidden Veggie Strawberry Cheesecake Smoothie (page 72), where it provides a nutritional boost without a detectable flavor. Yum!

Greek Yogurt: Don't let anyone lead you to believe Greek yogurt isn't keto-friendly! Plain unsweetened Greek yogurt is an amazing keto-friendly snack: not only low in carbs and calories, but also full of protein. I love to use it in keto baking to help my muffins and cakes get nice and fluffy.

Keto Sweeteners (Lakanto, Swerve, and equivalents): As you may have guessed, any kind of nutritive sweetener (a sweetener with calories) is going to be filled with carbohydrates. This includes table sugar, coconut sugar, dates, and honey. They spike your insulin and are not keto-friendly.

There are several non-nutritive sweeteners on the market now and you really get to choose whichever one works for you. They all taste sweet, but some are better than others. I would encourage you to try several and find one that you prefer.

My favorites are the brands Swerve (an erythritol and stevia blend) and Lakanto (an erythritol and monkfruit blend). They have a great taste and they measure one-for-one as a sugar replacement. These brands can be hard to find in countries outside of the US, but thanks to websites like Amazon, these types of keto products are becoming more and more available. If you cannot find Swerve or Lakanto, there are other brands that are very similar.

Xanthan Gum: This is probably the one ingredient you are giving a side-eye to, but don't let the name make you turn up your nose just yet! Xanthan gum is a thickener and emulsifier—think of it as the cornstarch of the keto world. (It can be found in a lot of premade foods you buy at the grocery store. Foods like cream cheese, ice cream, soups, and sauces.) I find mine at Walmart in the baking aisle. Once you buy a package, you will likely not need to buy it again until it expires as we use very little in the recipes but it makes a big impact on texture with very few carbs!

A Quick Note on Ground Beef

For all of the recipes in this book, I use 80/20 ground beef. This means the beef is 80 percent lean and 20 percent fat. I find this grind to be much more flavorful and delicious, and because of its higher fat content there is no need to add oil while cooking. If you want to use a leaner beef, say 93/7, some of the recipes, such as the Beef Taco Cups on page 180, may need a little oil to brown the ground beef without sticking.

My Go-To Equipment

Baking Sheets: I love to keep on hand rimmed baking sheets in various sizes. They are perfect for roasting meats and vegetables, sheet pan meals, and, of course, cookies!

Enameled Cast-Iron Pots (Dutch Oven): Anytime I make a soup, stew, or chili, you will find me using a Dutch oven. This heavy-duty pot will last a lifetime and should be in every home cook's kitchen.

Food Scale: When it comes to tracking your food, the more accurate you can be, the better. I weigh all of my calorie-dense foods on a food scale just to be sure I am eating the correct portion. This includes foods like cheese, nuts, meat, fats, and dressings.

Food Serving Scoops: I use these to perfectly portion my biscuits, cookies, meatballs, and muffins. I use a 3-tablespoon scoop for my biscuits and muffins, and I use a 2-tablespoon scoop for cookies and meatballs.

Meat Thermometer: One of the most important tools in my kitchen is a probe meat thermometer. There is no shame in using one to make sure your meat is perfectly cooked! I insert the probe into the center of the piece of meat, being sure to not go all of the way through. Chicken should be cooked to 165°F. Pork roasts and chops are safe to eat at 145°F (and in my opinion, that is when pork is the juiciest). For whole cuts of beef, 120°F is rare, 125°F is medium-rare, 130°F is medium, 145°F is medium-well, and 150°F is well done.

Silicone Baking Mats: I have silicone baking mats that fit all of the sizes of my baking sheets. I use these in place of foil or parchment paper sometimes for nonstick cooking without added oil.

Vegetable Spiralizer: These days, you can buy premade veggie noodles at many grocery stores. Noodles made from cucumber, yellow squash, zucchini, and other keto-friendly vegetables are easy alternatives to pasta. But making vegetables into noodles at home is so easy with one of these contraptions—not to mention, it'll save you money! Use a spiralizer to make my French Onion Chicken Zoodle Skillet on page 162.

KETO ON THE GO

Tips for Eating Out or Going on Vacation

As keto has grown in popularity, so, too, have the keto options at most restaurants—but sticking to the plan can still be tough if you're not in your own kitchen or traveling with unfamiliar food options nearby. Here are a few tips that will help you make the best choice anytime you are on the go.

Protein and vegetables will almost always be available. Choose grilled chicken or fish over breaded. Skip the rice and beans and add extra vegetables. Skip the bun and fries and have that burger over greens as a salad or in a lettuce wrap.

Don't be afraid to make substitutions. Believe me, your server has heard just about any substitution request you can think of, and kitchens are used to it! If that pasta dish with a creamy sauce and chicken is calling your name, think creatively so you can make the best choice for your goals. Replace the pasta with broccoli and have the sauce on the side.

Check the calorie count (but take it with a grain of salt). Many restaurants are sharing their calorie counts with their patrons, either on the menus or on their websites. Just be aware that restaurants usually do not weigh or measure portions, especially calorie-dense foods like cheese, nuts, dressings, and butter. You can almost guarantee the calorie count they post on their menu is less than what you are served. I like to estimate I am served 30 percent more calories than they post just to be on the safe side.

Think twice about the keto option. Sometimes the keto option isn't the best choice for your weight loss goals—so be sure to think about calories and not just carbs. Sometimes a big salad that looks to be keto-friendly can be over 1,000 calories! In instances like these, we can choose something a little more calorie-conscious and possibly eat a few more carbs that day, or take half of the dish to-go and save it for another meal.

Skip all the extra calories. Appetizers, drinks, desserts, chips, and bread baskets can add thousands of calories to a meal. Also, watch out for rich sauces and dressings. Ask for it on the side so you can have better portion control or skip it.

Plan it as an exception meal. Don't think you can never have an amazing meal at a restaurant ever again. Eating takeout or at a restaurant is really nice sometimes and I would never discourage anyone from doing so occasionally. Another option is to plan it as your exception meal and go all out! Don't let it turn into a slippery slope of off-plan eating all weekend, though. After these meals just get right back on track with your new normal.

When traveling, book accommodations with a kitchen. This is a great tip not only for saving money, but it will help keep you from having to eat out for every meal while on vacation.

Pack keto-friendly snacks. Road trips can be intimidating when you realize you have to worry about what and where you are going to eat! I like to pack my own food so I don't need to worry. I pack foods that are good cold, such as cooked bacon, hard-boiled eggs, nuts, cheese, and salami.

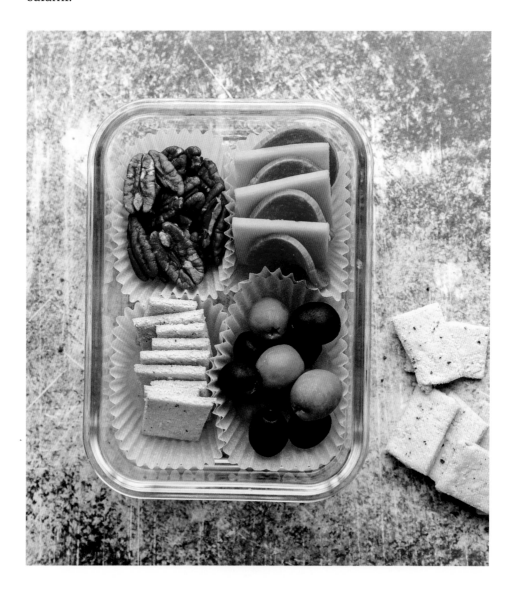

Part II:

THE RECIPES

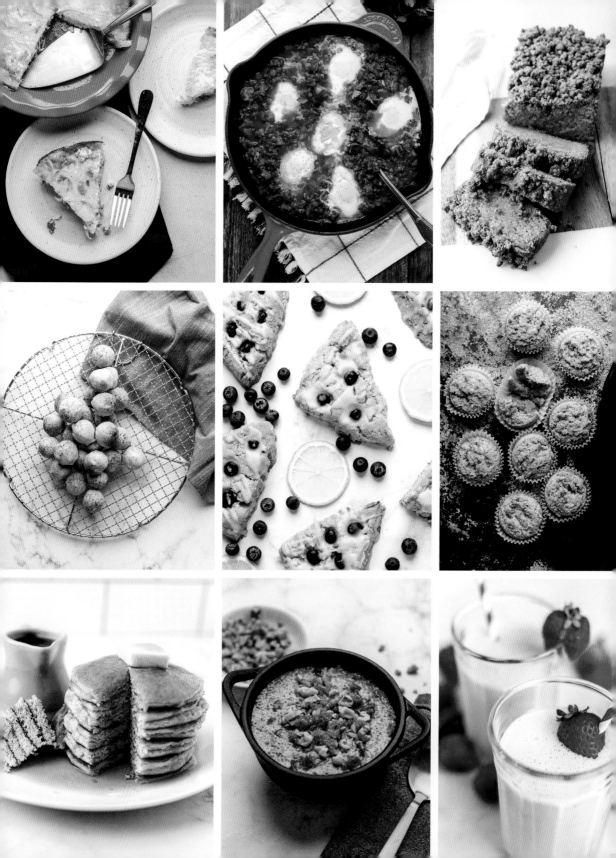

BREAKFAST

SAUCY CHORIZO EGGS IN PURGATORY

A dish of eggs poached in a tomato-based sauce, Eggs in Purgatory is a nearly effortless dish that is sure to impress—it's perfect for brunch or even a light dinner. This super-easy three-ingredient version is packed with flavor thanks to the magical ingredients, salsa and chorizo!

Prep Time: 5 minutes | Cook Time: 15 minutes | Total Time: 20 Minutes

1 pound ground chorizo

3 cups salsa of choice (choose one with minimal carbs)

6 large eggs

Small handful chopped fresh cilantro, for garnish (optional)

1. In a large-sized heavy-bottomed skillet with a lid, cook the chorizo over medium-high heat, breaking it up with a spoon, until browned and cooked through—about 8 minutes.

2. Stir in the salsa. Using a wooden spoon or spatula, make 6 wells in the mixture and crack an egg into each well.

3. Reduce the heat to medium and cover the skillet with a lid. Cook for 15 minutes or until the whites of the eggs are set and the yolks are still runny (depending on your desired doneness). Note that if you bring your eggs to room temperature before cracking them into the skillet, they may cook much faster. Garnish with cilantro if you like.

Makes 6 servings | Per serving: Calories: 337, Fat: 24g, Protein: 17g, Total CARBS: 7g, Fiber: 4g

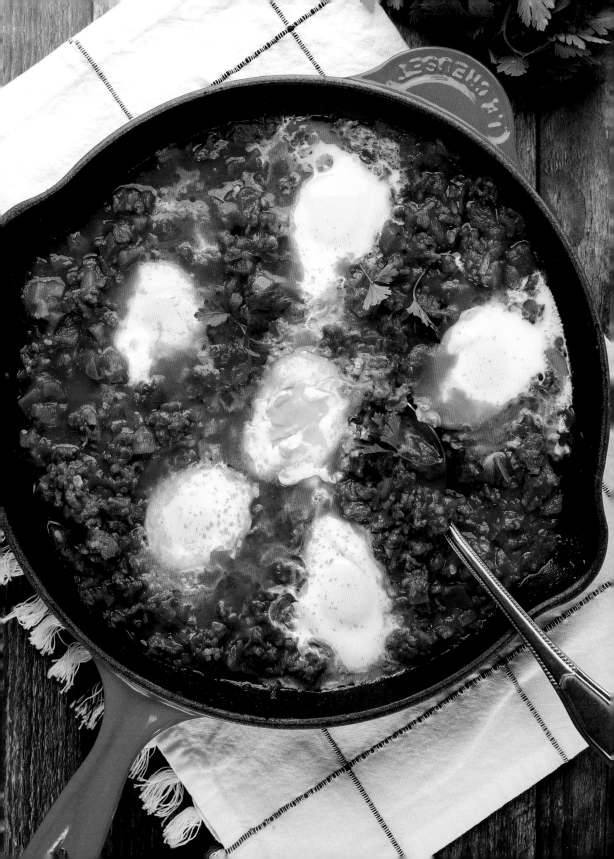

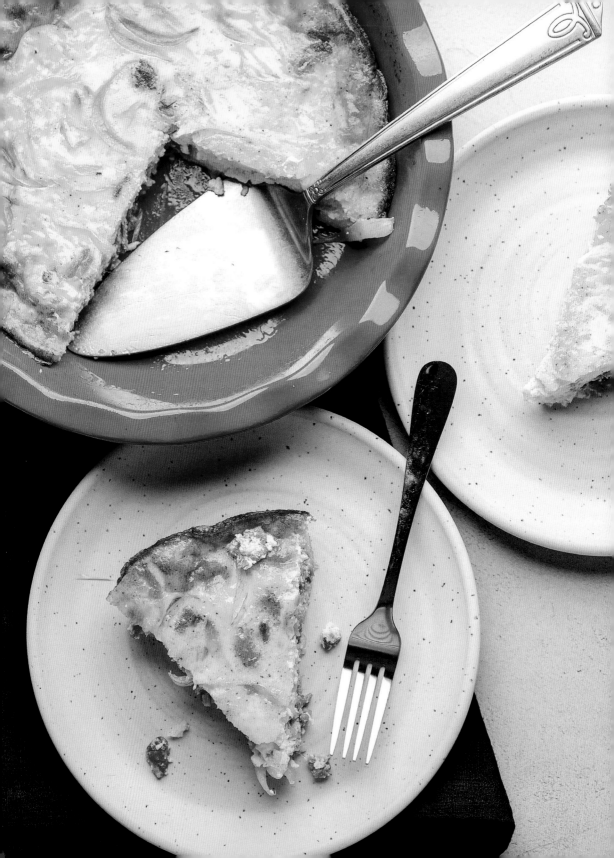

CRUSTLESS QUICHE LORRAINE

One of my family's favorite recipes is this crustless quiche, but they call it bacon pie! I've made so many variations of this over the years and they are always winners for breakfast or even dinner.

Prep Time: 10 minutes | Cook Time: 45 minutes | Total Time: 55 minutes

8 slices thick bacon, diced

½ white onion, sliced thin

6 large eggs

1½ cups half-and-half

½ teaspoon kosher salt

¼ teaspoon freshly ground
   black pepper

¼ teaspoon nutmeg

¼ teaspoon cayenne pepper

1½ cups shredded Swiss
   cheese

1. Preheat the oven to 375°F and grease a pie plate with butter or cooking spray.

2. In a large skillet over medium-high heat, cook the bacon and onion together until the bacon is crispy and the onions are soft and browned, about 15 minutes. Remove from the pan to a paper towel–lined plate and set aside.

3. In a large mixing bowl, combine the eggs, half-and-half, salt, pepper, nutmeg, and cayenne pepper. Beat with a whisk until well combined.

4. Stir the cheese, bacon, and caramelized onions into the mixing bowl with the eggs until well combined. Pour the mixture into the prepared pie plate and bake for 45 minutes or until the center is set.

Makes 1 quiche; 6 servings | Per serving: Calories: 334, Fat: 27g, Protein: 19g, Total CARBS: 5g, Fiber: 0g

CALIFORNIA SHEET PAN OMELETTE

When you want to make omelettes for a crowd, break out the sheet pan! This nutritious breakfast will keep you entertaining instead of manning the stovetop for hours.

Prep Time: 8 minutes | Cook Time: 25 minutes | Total Time: 33 minutes

12 large eggs

½ cup half-and-half

1 teaspoon kosher salt

½ teaspoon black pepper

2 cups shredded cheddar cheese

4 ounces mushrooms, sliced

Optional Toppings

Crumbled bacon

Sliced avocado

Diced tomato

1. Preheat the oven to 350°F. Line the bottom of a 9 × 13–inch rimmed sheet pan with parchment paper and grease with oil or cooking spray.

2. In a large mixing bowl, whisk together the eggs, half-and-half, salt, and pepper until the mixture is a pale yellow color.

3. Pour the egg mixture into the prepared sheet pan and top with the shredded cheese and sliced mushrooms. Bake in the oven for 25 minutes, until the eggs are completely set. Slice into 8 equal servings and serve topped with your favorite omelette toppings.

Makes 8 servings | Per serving: Calories: 269, Fat: 23g, Protein: 17g, Total CARBS: 1g, Fiber: 0g

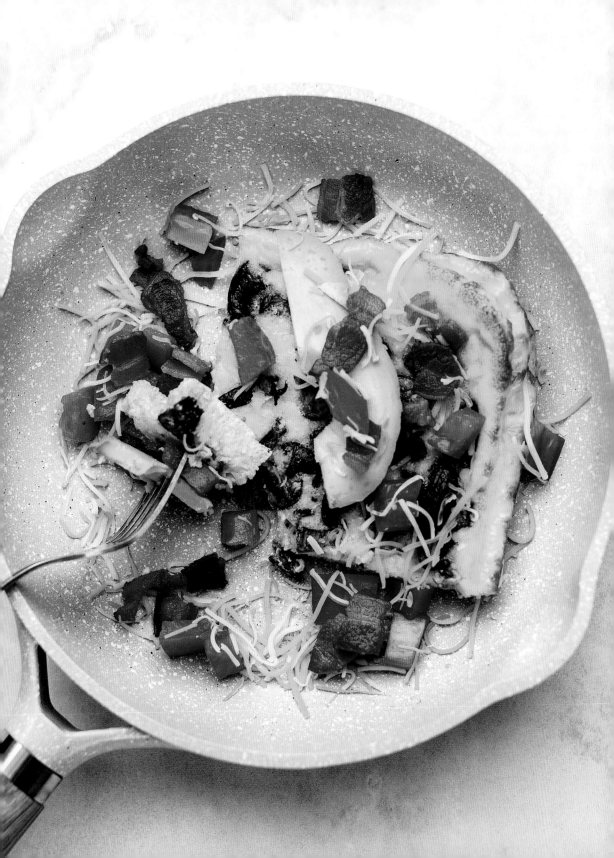

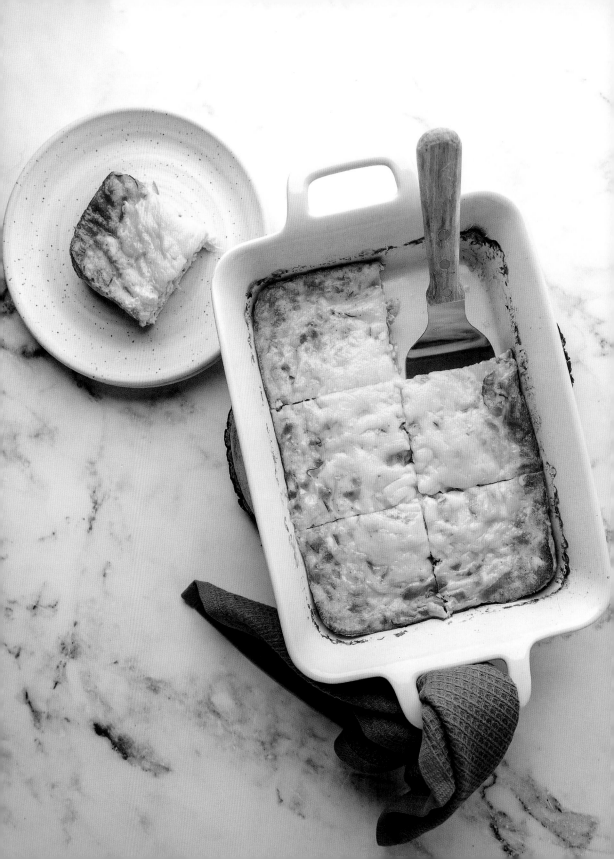

HAM AND SWISS BREAKFAST CASSEROLE

This brunch-friendly recipe easily doubles for large gatherings! Simply double the ingredients and bake in a 9 × 13–inch casserole dish until the center is set.

Prep Time: 5 minutes | Cook Time: 45 minutes | Total Time: 50 minutes

10 large eggs

1 cup half-and-half

¼ teaspoon ground nutmeg

½ teaspoon kosher salt

12 oz cooked ham, diced

2 cups shredded Swiss cheese, divided

1. Preheat the oven to 350°F and grease a 3-quart casserole dish with butter or cooking spray.

2. In a large mixing bowl, combine the eggs, half-and-half, nutmeg, and salt. Whisk until well combined. Stir in the ham and the 1½ cups of the cheese and pour into the prepared casserole dish. Top with the remaining ½ cup of cheese.

3. Bake for 45 minutes, until the center is set.

Makes 6 servings | Per serving: Calories: 373, Fat: 25g, Protein: 31g, Total CARBS: 5g, Fiber: 0g

SAUSAGE AND RADISH BREAKFAST HASH

Yes, a hash that is light on calories and carbs thanks to the humble radish! Trust me, you are going to make this a staple in your breakfast rotation.

Prep Time: 15 minutes | Cook Time: 15 minutes | Total Time: 30 minutes

1½ pounds radishes (tops removed and diced into ½-inch-sized pieces)

2 teaspoons kosher salt

2 tablespoons avocado oil

1 pound ground breakfast sausage (casings removed if using links)

½ cup diced onion

½ cup diced green bell pepper

½ cup diced red bell pepper

3 garlic cloves, minced

6 large eggs

1. Place the diced radishes and salt in a medium-sized pot and cover the radishes with water. Bring to a boil over high heat. Let cook until the radishes are almost tender, about 5 minutes. Drain the liquid and set the radishes aside.

2. Heat the avocado oil in a large skillet over medium-high heat. Add the sausage, onion, and bell pepper. Sauté, breaking up the sausage with a wooden spoon, until the sausage is cooked through, about 10 minutes. Stir in the garlic and radishes and cook for 5 minutes more.

3. While the hash is cooking, prepare the eggs to your liking. If you like yours sunny-side up, like I do, heat a small or medium nonstick skillet with a tight-fitting lid over medium heat. Crack 3 eggs in the pan and cover with the lid. Cook until the white is set, about 5 minutes; carefully remove to a plate and repeat with the remaining eggs.

4. Serve the hash topped with sunny-side up eggs.

Makes 6 servings; 1 cup hash plus 1 egg per serving | Per serving: Calories: 388, Fat: 29g, Protein: 23g, Total CARBS: 5g, Fiber: 2g

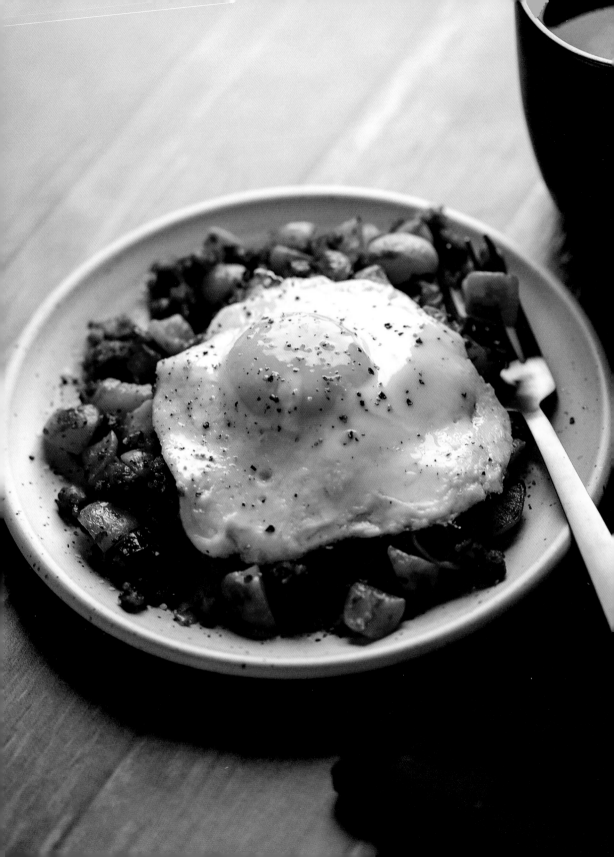

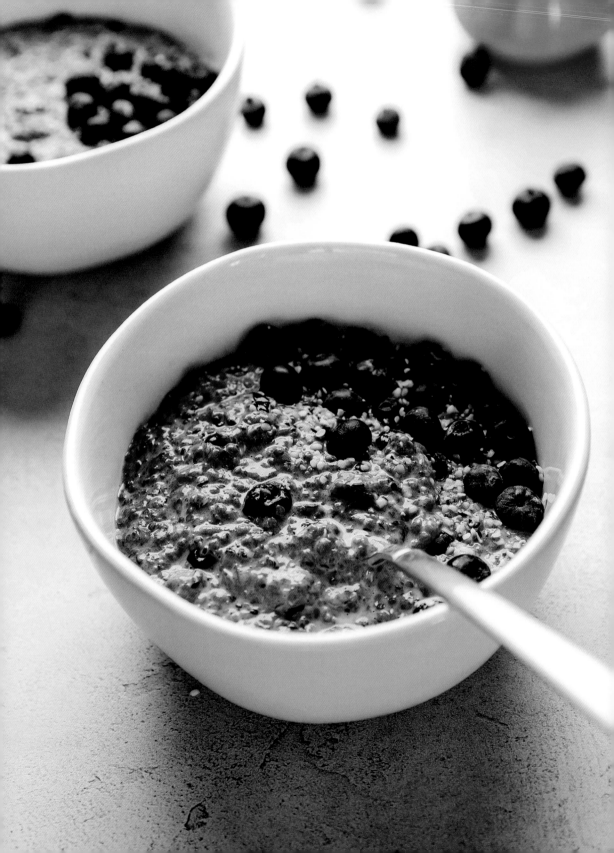

BLUEBERRY NOATMEAL

This no-oat oatmeal recipe can be made ahead, and having this delicious breakfast on hand during the week makes busy mornings so much easier and less stressful.

Prep Time: 5 minutes | Cook Time: 5 minutes | Total Time: 10 minutes

¾ cup hemp hearts

3 tablespoons granulated sweetener

1 tablespoon chia seeds

2 teaspoons cinnamon

2 teaspoons vanilla

1 cup water

¾ cup heavy cream

1 cup blueberries

1. In a medium-sized saucepan over medium heat, combine all of the ingredients. Cook for 5–8 minutes until thick, stirring occasionally.

2. Divide the cooked "oatmeal" among 4 bowls and serve. Or divide it among 4 airtight containers with lids, let cool, and refrigerate for up to 1 week. To reheat, microwave on high for 1 minute or until heated through.

Makes 4 servings; ⅔ cup per serving | Per serving: Calories: 371, Fat: 34g, Protein: 11g, Total CARBS: 9g, Fiber: 4g

BROWN SUGAR CHIA PUDDING WITH WALNUTS

At virtually zero carbs, chia seeds are a nutritional powerhouse. They make for a very filling sugar-free breakfast that is easy to prep ahead of time. This chia pudding stores in the refrigerator in an airtight container for up to one week.

Prep Time: 5 minutes | Cook Time: 5 minutes | Total Time: 10 minutes

½ cup chia seeds

⅓ cup brown sugar sweetener, more for garnish

½ teaspoon cinnamon

¼ teaspoon kosher salt

1 cup water

¾ cup half-and-half

½ teaspoon vanilla extract

½ cup chopped walnuts, more for garnish

1. In a medium-sized saucepan over medium heat, combine all of the ingredients except the walnuts. Stir frequently so as not to scorch the bottom of the pan. Cook for about 5 minutes or until your ingredients begin to thicken and the chia seeds soften.

2. Divide into ½-cup servings and garnish with walnuts and extra brown sugar sweetener.

Makes 4 servings; ½ cup per serving | Per serving: Calories: 290, Fat: 23g, Protein: 8g, Total CARBS: 16g, Fiber: 11g

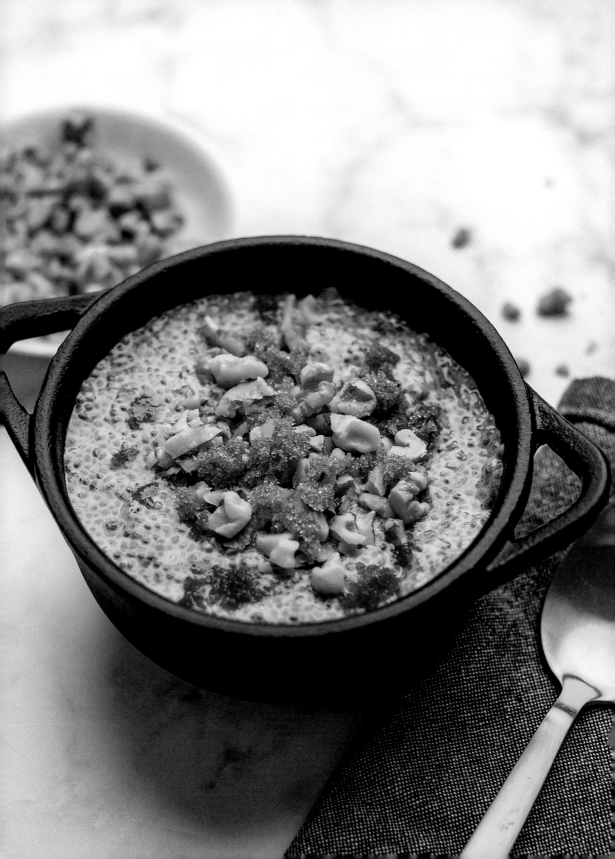

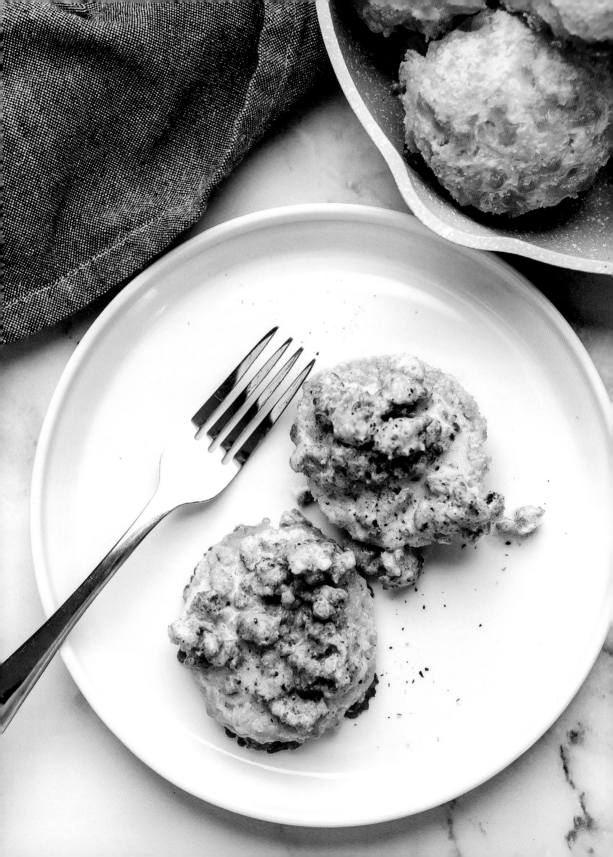

CHEDDAR BISCUITS AND SAUSAGE GRAVY

I love a good biscuit but I have to say these keto-friendly cheddar biscuits are so amazing, I would make these even if I weren't eating keto. Paired with the sausage gravy, this hearty breakfast is the perfect start to the day.

Prep Time: 10 minutes | Cook Time: 15 minutes | Total Time: 25 minutes

Cheddar Biscuits

2 cups almond flour

1 cup shredded cheddar cheese

¼ teaspoon baking powder

¼ teaspoon kosher salt

4 large eggs

Sausage Gravy

½ pound ground pork sausage

1 cup chicken broth

1 cup half-and-half

½ teaspoon xanthan gum

Salt and pepper to taste

Makes 6 servings; 1 biscuit and ½ cup gravy per serving | Per serving: Calories: 526, Fat: 44g, Protein: 25g, Total CARBS: 10g, Fiber: 4g

1. Preheat the oven to 400°F and line a small baking sheet with parchment paper or a silicone baking mat.

2. For the biscuits, stir together the almond flour, cheddar cheese, baking powder, and salt in a large mixing bowl until well combined. Stir in the eggs until fully incorporated. The batter will be thick and hold its shape. Using a spoon or 3-tablespoon scoop, divide the batter evenly into 6 rounds on the parchment-lined baking sheet. Pat into discs and bake for 15 minutes, until golden brown. Remove the biscuits to a wire rack to cool slightly.

3. For the sausage gravy, in a large skillet over medium-high heat, cook the sausage, breaking it up with a wooden spoon, until it is browned and cooked through, about 8 minutes. Stir in the chicken broth, half-and-half, and xanthan gum. Bring to a boil, then reduce the heat to a simmer and cook until the gravy thickens, about 5 minutes. Season with salt and pepper to taste.

4. Serve the biscuits with the hot gravy.

CINNAMON CRUNCH BREAD

When your non-keto dad doesn't want to share a piece of this bread with anyone, you know you've got a winner on your hands. Store the bread in an airtight container in the refrigerator for up to one week or keep frozen for up to two months!

Prep Time: 10 minutes | Cook Time: 35 minutes | Total Time: 45 minutes

2 cups almond flour

½ teaspoon kosher salt

½ cup granulated sweetener

1 teaspoon baking soda

3 large eggs, beaten

¼ cup butter, melted

Crumble Topping

⅓ cup almond flour

2 tablespoons granulated sweetener

1 teaspoon cinnamon

2 tablespoons melted butter

1. Preheat the oven to 350°F and grease an 8 × 4–inch loaf pan with butter or cooking spray.

2. In a large mixing bowl, stir together the dry ingredients until well combined. Stir in the beaten eggs and melted butter. The batter will be thick.

3. Spread the batter into the greased loaf pan and bake for 35 minutes. Bread will not be cooked through.

4. Meanwhile, in a small mixing bowl, stir together the ingredients for the crumble topping until well combined.

5. At 35 minutes, use a spoon to top the bread evenly with the crumble. Place back in the oven for 20 minutes, until the crumble browns and a toothpick inserted in the center of the loaf comes out clean. Let cool in the pan for 20 minutes before cutting into 8 (1-inch) slices and serving.

Makes 1 loaf; 8 servings | Per serving: Calories: 293, Fat: 27g, Protein: 9g, Total CARBS: 6g, Fiber: 4g

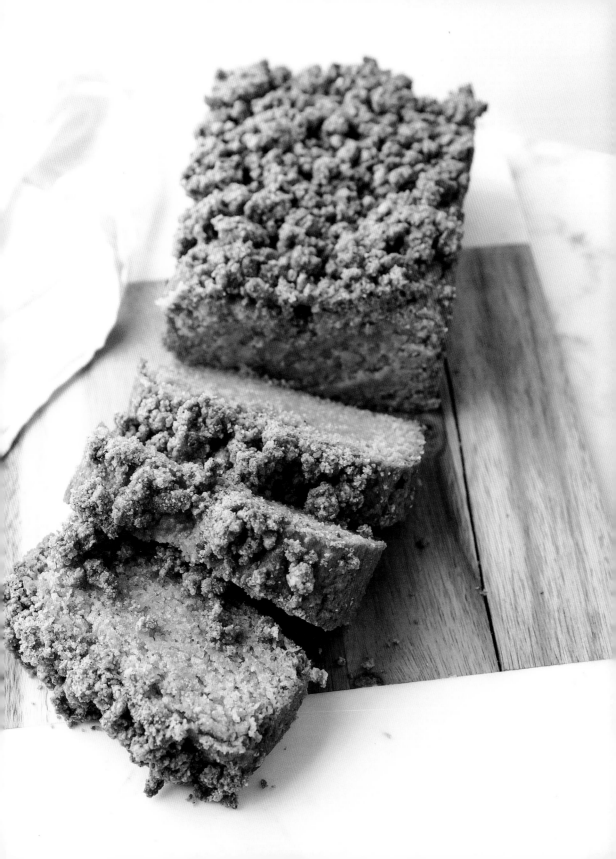

LEMON BLUEBERRY SCONES

I don't know about you, but I was never wild about scones before because they can be very crumbly and dry. Enter my Lemon Blueberry Scones. *These* scones are packed with fruity flavor and perfectly moist.

Prep Time: 10 minutes | Cook Time: 25 minutes | Total Time: 35 minutes

3 cups almond flour

½ cup granulated sweetener

1 tablespoon lemon zest

1½ teaspoons baking soda

½ teaspoon kosher salt

4 tablespoons cold butter, cut into cubes

2 large eggs

3 tablespoons lemon juice, divided

⅓ cup blueberries

½ cup powdered sweetener

1. Preheat the oven to 350°F and line a half sheet pan with parchment paper or a silicone baking mat.

2. In a large bowl, stir together the almond flour, granulated sweetener, lemon zest, baking soda, and kosher salt until well combined. Add the cold butter. Using your hands, forks, or a pastry cutter, incorporate the butter into the almond flour until it forms pea-sized crumbles.

3. In a separate small bowl, beat together the eggs and 2 tablespoons of the lemon juice. Gently stir the egg mixture into the dry mixture until just combined.

4. Turn the dough out onto a work surface and form into a disk about 1 inch thick. Cut into 8 triangles and arrange on the baking sheet. Press the blueberries evenly into the scones.

5. Bake for 20–25 minutes, until a toothpick inserted in the center comes out clean. Cool completely on a wire rack before applying the glaze.

6. Stir together the remaining 1 tablespoon lemon juice and the powdered sweetener in a small bowl until well combined. If needed, thin the glaze with water, 1 teaspoon at a time, to get your desired consistency. Drizzle the glaze evenly over each scone.

Makes 8 scones; 1 per serving | Per serving: Calories: 328, Fat: 30g, Protein: 11g, Total CARBS: 9g, Fiber: 5g

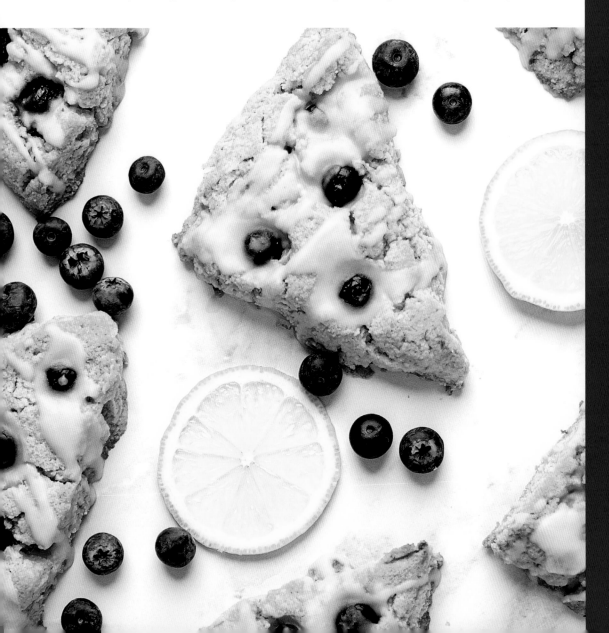

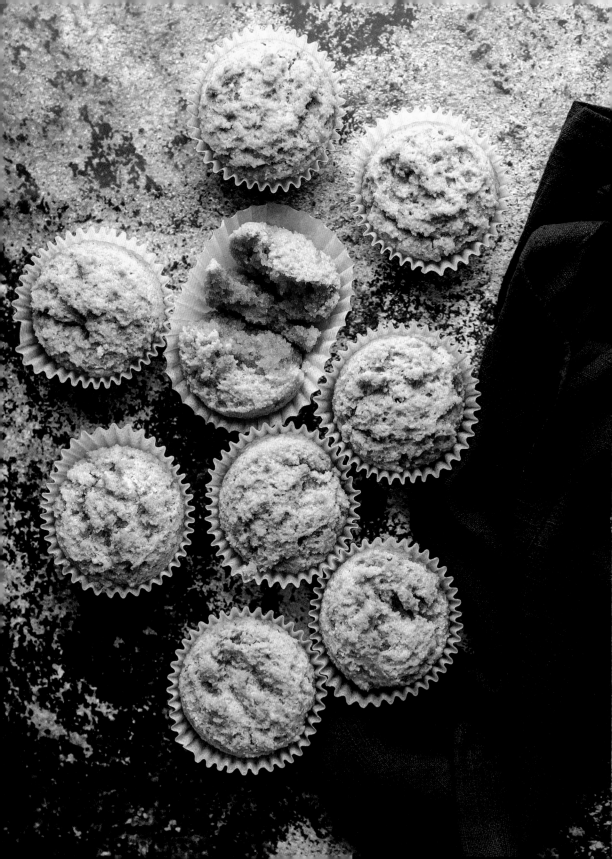

MAPLE VANILLA MUFFINS

Maple flavoring is such a great product and gives people enjoying a keto lifestyle more options when it comes to baking. You can find it in most major grocery stores. Freeze these muffins on a plate or sheet pan, then transfer to a freezer bag or bowl so you can enjoy them for up to two months!

Prep Time: 10 minutes | Cook Time: 15 minutes | Total Time: 25 minutes

2½ cups almond flour

⅓ cup granulated sweetener

1 teaspoon baking soda

½ teaspoon kosher salt

3 large eggs, beaten

¼ cup melted butter

1 teaspoon vanilla extract

1 teaspoon maple extract

1. Preheat the oven to 350°F. Line a 12-well muffin tin with paper liners and spray with cooking spray.

2. In a large mixing bowl, stir together the dry ingredients until well combined. Stir in the beaten eggs, melted butter, vanilla extract, and maple extract until well combined. The batter will be thick.

3. Divide the batter evenly between the muffin cups and bake for 15 minutes or until the tops of the muffins are lightly browned and a toothpick inserted in the center comes out clean. Cool in the pan for 10 minutes.

Makes 12 muffins; 1 per serving | Per serving: Calories: 194, Fat: 18g, Protein: 7g, Total CARBS: 4g, Fiber: 3g

LEMON POPPY SEED LOAF

Quick breads were always a staple in my home as a child. I am excited to be able to share my love of these easy recipes with my children and continue the tradition. Store the bread in an airtight container in the refrigerator for up to one week or keep frozen for up to two months.

Prep Time: 5 minutes | Cook Time: 40 minutes | Total Time: 45 minutes

2 cups almond flour

1 tablespoon poppy seeds

½ cup granulated sweetener

Zest of a whole lemon

1 teaspoon baking soda

½ teaspoon kosher salt

3 large eggs, beaten

¼ cup butter, melted

3 tablespoons lemon juice

1. Preheat the oven to 350°F and grease the inside of an 8 × 4–inch loaf pan with butter or cooking spray.

2. Combine the dry ingredients in a large mixing bowl until well combined. Stir in the eggs, butter, and lemon juice.

3. Spread the batter into the prepared loaf pan and bake for 40 minutes or until the top is lightly browned and a toothpick inserted in the center comes out clean. Cool completely in the pan before cutting into 8 (1-inch) slices and serving.

Makes 1 loaf; 8 servings | Per serving: Calories: 246, Fat: 22g, Protein: 8g, Total CARBS: 6g, Fiber: 3g

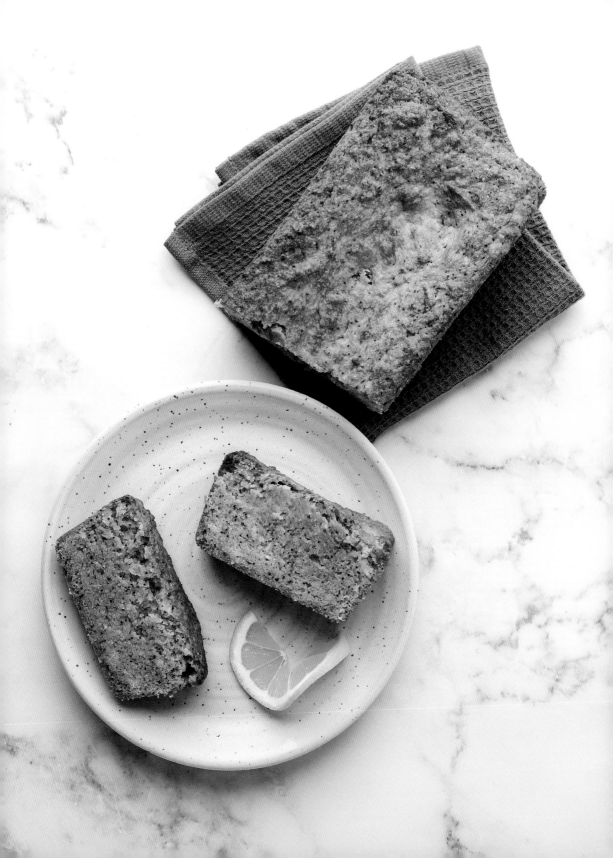

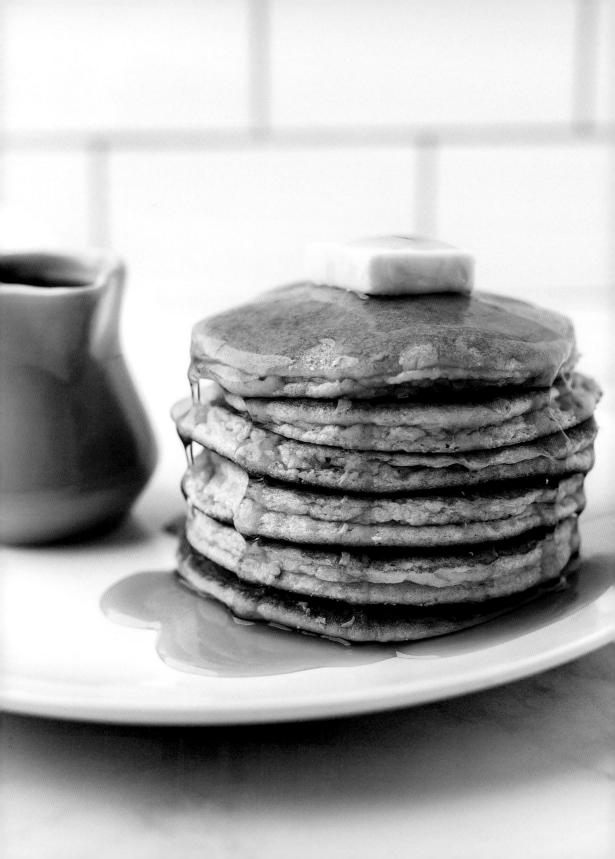

FLUFFY SUNDAY MORNING PANCAKES

Making fluffy pancakes on Sunday morning is a tradition I can get behind, especially if they are keto like these! The secret to making them thick and airy is separating the eggs and whipping the whites separately. In this recipe, you'll use just one of the yolks. Save the reserved yolk to add to another recipe!

Prep Time: 10 minutes | Cook Time: 20 minutes | Total Time: 30 minutes

1 cup almond flour

1 tablespoon granulated sweetener

1 teaspoon baking powder

2 large eggs, separated

½ cup unsweetened almond milk

1 teaspoon vanilla

1. In a large mixing bowl, stir together the almond flour, sweetener, and baking powder until well combined. Stir in 1 egg yolk, the almond milk, and vanilla. (Reserve the other egg yolk for another purpose.) Set aside the batter.

2. In a small mixing bowl, beat the egg whites using a hand mixer until stiff white peaks form. Fold the whites into the pancake batter. Let the pancake batter sit for 5 minutes to thicken.

3. Grease a nonstick griddle or large nonstick skillet with cooking spray or oil and heat over medium heat. Pour ¼-cup portions of the batter into the skillet or on the griddle and let cook until bubbles start to form on the edges, about 3 minutes, then carefully flip and continue cooking until slightly golden, about 2 minutes. Repeat with the remaining batter. Serve with your favorite keto toppings (I like butter and sugar-free syrup).

Makes 4 servings; 2 pancakes per serving | Per serving, without toppings: Calories: 204, Fat: 17g, Protein: 9g, Total CARBS: 6g, Fiber: 3g

HIDDEN VEGGIE STRAWBERRY CHEESECAKE SMOOTHIE

Do not be alarmed by the presence of cauliflower in this smoothie! It is truly undetectable. A smoothie is the perfect opportunity to sneak some veggies into your kids' diet (or your own)! I recommend Premier Protein brand's Vanilla Milkshake Protein Powder, but feel free to use your favorite one. Look for one with minimal carbs per serving.

Prep Time: 5 minutes | Total Time: 5 minutes

2 cups ice cubes

2 cups unsweetened almond milk

1 cup frozen cauliflower rice

1 cup unsweetened frozen strawberries

½ cup powdered sweetener

8 ounces cream cheese, cubed

2 scoops low-carb vanilla protein powder

Combine all of the ingredients in a high-speed blender and blend until smooth. Divide evenly among 4 cups. Enjoy immediately.

Makes 4 servings | Per serving: Calories: 324, Fat: 23g, Protein: 20g, Total CARBS: 10g, Fiber: 3g

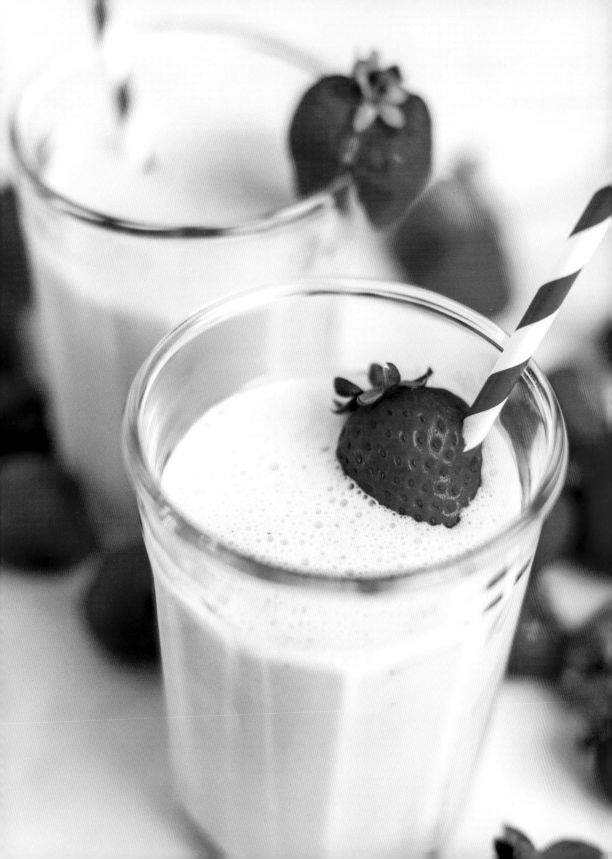

CINNAMON ROLL ENERGY BITES

These little bites pack a flavor and energy punch. Just what you need for an early morning pick-me-up! Energy bites are high in satiating fat, so they're great for keeping hunger under control. They are small but calorie-dense so you can adjust your serving size to fit your own goals. If you have a ½-tablespoon cookie scoop, you can use it to get heaping scoops that are the perfect size for this recipe.

Prep Time: 15 minutes | Chill Time: 30 minutes | Total Time: 45 minutes

2 cups almond flour

4 tablespoons granulated sweetener

2 teaspoons cinnamon, plus extra for sprinkling

Pinch of kosher salt

½ cup butter, melted

2 teaspoons vanilla extract

9 ounces sugar-free white chocolate chips

1 tablespoon coconut oil

1. Line a half sheet pan with parchment paper.

2. Stir together the almond flour, sweetener, cinnamon, and salt in a medium-sized mixing bowl until combined. Mix in the butter and vanilla extract and stir until a thick batter is formed.

3. Scoop out the mixture into 1-tablespoon-sized rounds and place on the lined cookie sheet, evenly spaced. With your hands, roll into balls and arrange on the prepared sheet pan. You should end up with 24 balls. Place the energy bites into the freezer for 20 minutes.

4. Combine the chocolate chips and the coconut oil in a medium-sized heat-proof bowl. Fill a saucepan halfway with water and bring to a simmer. Set the bowl of chocolate on the pan over the simmering water and cook, stirring frequently, until the chocolate is completely melted. Remove from the heat.

CREAM OF MUSHROOM AND CHICKEN SOUP WITH ROASTED GARLIC

The roasted garlic really elevates the flavor of this cream of mushroom soup without much additional effort.

Prep Time: 10 minutes | Cook Time: 45 minutes | Total Time: 55 minutes

5 garlic cloves, skin on

3 boneless, skinless chicken breasts

Salt and pepper

1 tablespoon unsalted butter

½ cup diced onion

8 ounces baby bella mushrooms, finely chopped

4 cups chicken broth

1 cup heavy cream

1 teaspoon xanthan gum

Fresh parsley leaves, for garnish (optional)

1. Preheat the oven to 350°F and lightly grease a rimmed baking sheet. Wrap the cloves of garlic in a small piece of aluminum foil.

2. Place the chicken breasts and the foil-wrapped garlic on the prepared baking sheet. Season both sides of the chicken with salt and pepper. Bake for 30 minutes, until the chicken's internal temperature is 165°F (tested using an instant read internal meat thermometer). Remove from the oven and let cool for 5 minutes, then chop the chicken into bite-sized pieces. Remove the garlic cloves from the foil. Set aside.

3. Melt the butter in a medium-sized heavy-bottomed pot over medium heat. Add the onion and season lightly with salt and pepper. Cook the onion, stirring occasionally, until translucent, about 5 minutes. Pop the individual garlic cloves from their skins and stir into the onions, gently chopping with a spoon to break up the cloves.

4. Stir in the mushrooms and season lightly with salt. Cook for 5 minutes more, stirring occasionally, until the mushrooms are tender

SOUPS AND STEWS

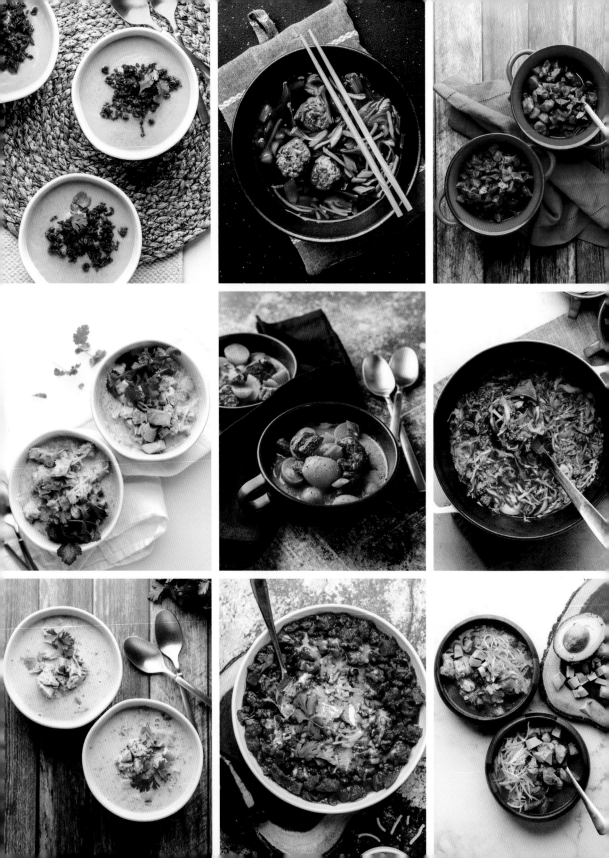

5. Dip each ball into the chocolate mixture and coat completely. Set back on the lined sheet tray. Continue with the remaining balls. Sprinkle with extra cinnamon if desired. Freeze for an additional 10 minutes. Keep refrigerated in an airtight container until ready to eat.

Makes 24 energy bites; 3 per serving | Per serving: Calories: 415, Fat: 37g, Protein: 6g, Total CARBS: 12g, Fiber: 10g

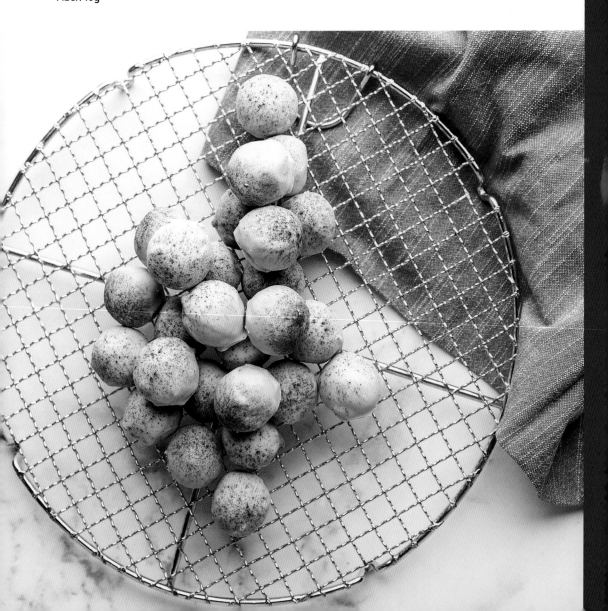

and lightly browned. Stir in the chicken broth, heavy cream, chicken, and xanthan gum. Bring to a boil, then reduce the heat to a simmer and cook for 5 minutes, until the soup has thickened slightly. Season with additional salt and pepper to taste. If you like, garnish each bowl with some fresh parsley.

Makes 4 servings; 1½ cups per serving | Per serving: Calories: 411, Fat: 30g, Protein: 33g, Total CARBS: 7g, Fiber: 2g

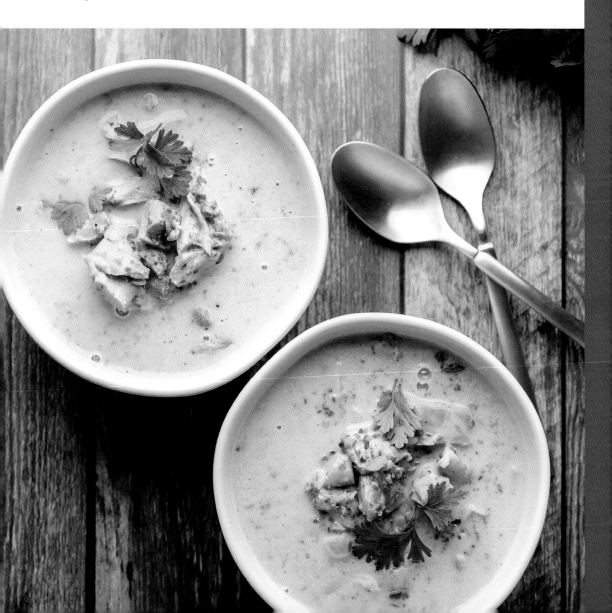

BUTTERNUT SQUASH AND ZUCCHINI SOUP WITH CRISPY CHORIZO

This creamy butternut squash soup is made into a complete meal with the addition of crispy chorizo. This one is sure to warm you up!

Prep Time: 10 minutes | Cook Time: 20 minutes | Total Time: 30 minutes

2 cups chicken broth

12 ounces butternut squash, peeled and cut into 1-inch chunks

3 medium zucchini (about 1½ pounds), ends removed and diced

1 (13.5-ounce) can full-fat coconut milk

Salt and pepper

1 pound ground chorizo

Fresh cilantro, for garnish (optional)

1. Heat the chicken broth in a medium-sized heavy-bottomed pot over high heat. Add the butternut squash and bring to a boil. Reduce the heat to a simmer, cover with a lid, and cook until the squash is fork tender, about 8 minutes.

2. Stir in the chopped zucchini and cook for 5 minutes more until the zucchini is fork tender.

3. Stir in the coconut milk. Use an immersion blender to puree the soup in the pot. (Alternatively, you can use a blender to puree the soup. You may need to work in batches depending on the size of your blender. Work carefully as the hot soup may splash.) Season with salt and pepper to taste.

4. While the soup is cooking, crisp the chorizo. In a large skillet over medium-high heat, cook the chorizo until browned and crispy, breaking up any clumps with a wooden spoon, about 8 minutes. Remove from the pan with a slotted spoon to a plate lined with paper towels and set aside.

5. Serve the soup in bowls topped with the crispy chorizo. If desired, garnish the soup with some fresh cilantro.

Makes 6 servings; 1¼ cups soup plus ⅓ cup chorizo per serving | Per serving: Calories: 396, Fat: 32g, Protein: 14g, Total CARBS: 15g, Fiber: 5g

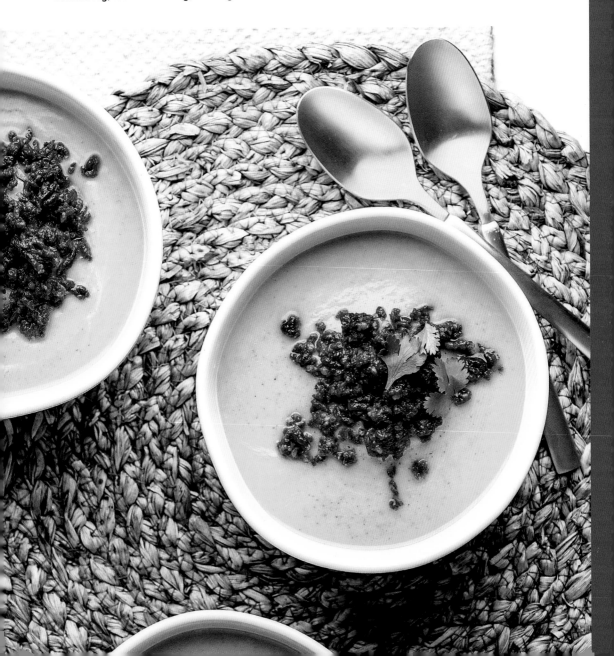

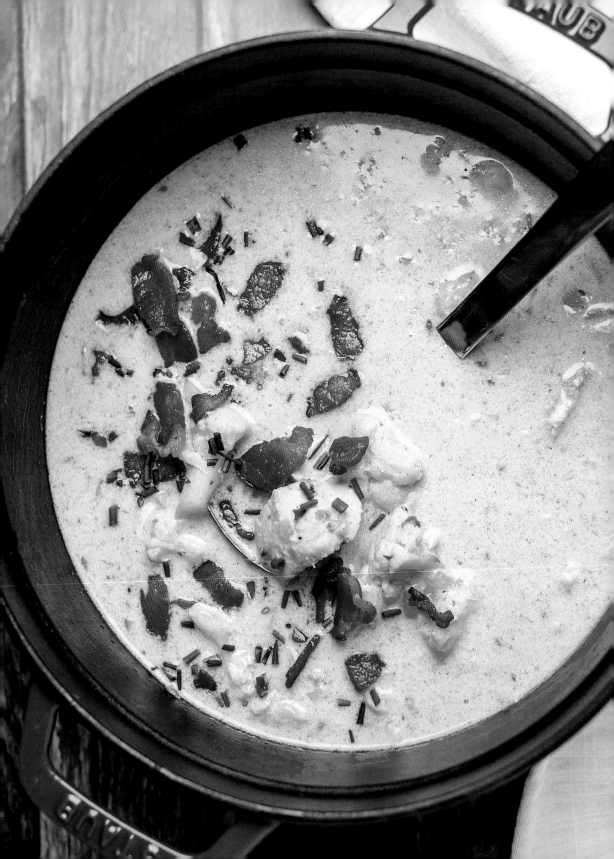

SALMON CHOWDER

A chowder can seem like it'll take time and effort to prepare, but I can assure you, this recipe cooks up so quickly and easily. The cauliflower and salmon cook in a jiff so you will be curled up with a warm bowl of soup in no time.

Prep Time: 10 minutes | Cook Time: 25 minutes | Total Time: 35 minutes

½ pound bacon, chopped

½ cup diced onion

2 garlic cloves, minced

12 ounces frozen cauliflower florets, thawed

3 cups chicken broth

1 cup heavy cream

1 pound boneless, skinless salmon, cut into 1-inch chunks

Salt and pepper to taste

Chopped fresh chives, for garnish (optional)

1. In a medium-sized heavy-bottomed pot over medium-high heat, cook the bacon until crispy, about 8 minutes. Remove with a slotted spoon and drain on a plate lined with paper towels. Set the bacon aside.

2. Reduce the heat to medium and remove all but 2 tablespoons of bacon fat from the pot. Stir in the onion and cook for about 5 minutes until translucent. Stir in the garlic and cook for 1 minute more until fragrant.

3. Stir in the cauliflower, chicken broth, heavy cream, and salmon. Cook until the salmon is cooked through, about 5 minutes. Adjust seasoning to taste.

4. Serve topped with reserved crispy bacon. If you like, garnish the soup with some chopped fresh chives.

Makes 6 servings; 1 cup per serving | Per serving: Calories: 429, Fat: 36g, Protein: 26g, Total CARBS: 6g, Fiber: 1g

SPICY POBLANO CHILI

This hearty chili is full of irresistible smoky flavor thanks to chipotle peppers in adobo sauce—I bet it'll win you over even if you aren't always a fan of spicy foods. If you've never had them, chipotles in adobo are smoked, dried jalapeño peppers that are rehydrated and canned in a tangy tomato sauce. They can be found in most grocery stores in the international aisles. If you are having trouble finding them, you can substitute with 3 tablespoons of diced and seeded jalapeños and a tablespoon of smoked paprika.

Prep Time: 10 minutes | Cook Time: 2 hours | Total Time: 2 hours, 10 minutes

1 tablespoon avocado oil

1 pound beef stew meat, cut into 1-inch cubes

Salt and pepper

½ cup diced onion

2 poblano peppers, seeded and chopped

3 garlic cloves, minced

½ pound ground chorizo

2 tablespoons tomato paste

2 tablespoons chili powder

3 chipotles in adobo, chopped

1 tablespoon onion powder

1 tablespoon cumin

1 (28-ounce) can fire-roasted diced tomatoes

1½ cups shredded cheddar cheese (optional)

Fresh cilantro, for garnish (optional)

1. Heat the avocado oil in a large-sized heavy-bottomed pot over high heat. Working in batches if necessary so you don't crowd the pan, add the stew meat and season with salt and pepper. Sear the stew meat for a couple minutes on all sides, until a brown crust forms. Remove to a plate and set aside.

2. Reduce the heat to medium and stir in the onion and poblano peppers. Cook for 5 minutes, until the onion is translucent. Stir in the minced garlic and cook for 1 minute more until fragrant. Add the ground chorizo and cook until browned, breaking up any clumps with a wooden spoon, about 6 minutes.

3. Stir in the tomato paste and remaining seasonings and cook for a few minutes, until fragrant. Stir in the roasted diced tomatoes and reserved beef stew meat. Cover with a lid and

simmer, stirring occasionally, for 90 minutes, or until the beef stew meat is fork tender. If you like, top the chili with shredded cheddar and fresh cilantro.

Makes 6 servings; 1 cup per serving | Per serving, without optional cheese topping: Calories: 412, Fat: 28g, Protein: 26g, Total CARBS: 15g, Fiber: 4g

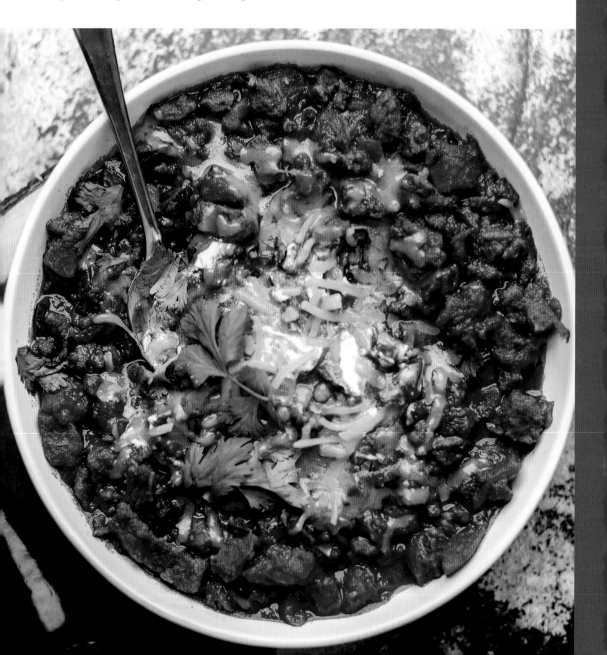

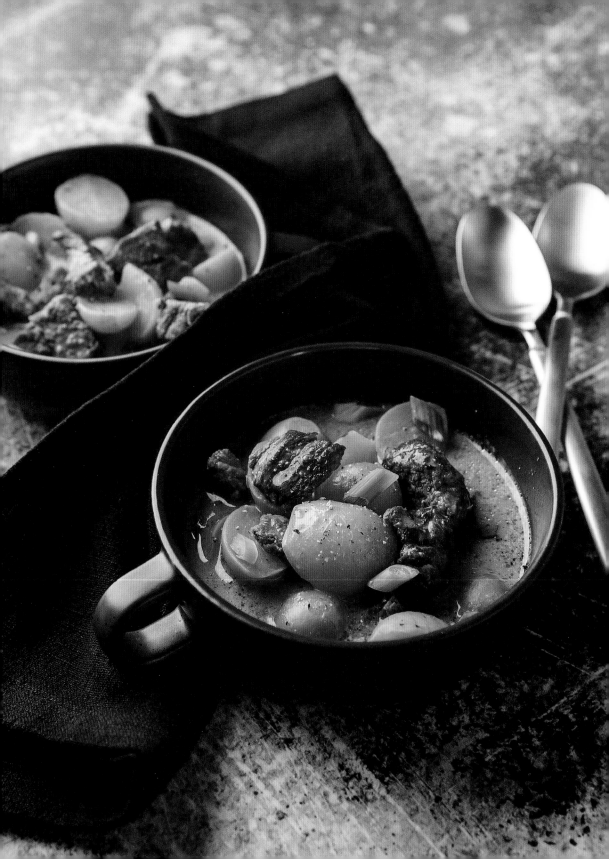

STEAK AND FAUXTATO SOUP

I kid you not, radishes are the new potatoes. This hearty soup brings all the appeal of meat and potatoes but clocks in at only 2 net carbs! (You can also see the magic of radishes in the Sausage and Radish Breakfast Hash on page 54.)

Prep Time: 10 minutes | Cook Time: 2 hours | Total Time: 2 hours, 10 minutes

2 tablespoons avocado oil

1½ pounds beef sirloin, cut into 1-inch cubes

½ teaspoon kosher salt

¼ teaspoon pepper

2 bunches red radishes, tops removed and halved (about 25 radishes)

1 teaspoon dried thyme

½ teaspoon garlic powder

½ teaspoon onion powder

32 ounces beef broth

½ teaspoon xanthan gum

½ cup heavy cream

Chopped green onions, for garnish (optional)

1. Heat the avocado oil in a large-sized heavy-bottomed pot over high heat. Add the beef and season with salt and pepper. Sear the beef for a couple minutes on all sides, until a brown crust forms.

2. Stir in the remaining ingredients except for the heavy cream. Bring to a simmer, cover with a lid, and cook for 1½ hours, until the beef is fork tender. Remove from the heat and stir in the heavy cream. Serve immediately topped with some chopped green onions if you like.

Makes 6 servings; 1½ cups per serving | Per serving: Calories: 383, Fat: 30g, Protein: 24g, Total CARBS: 3g, Fiber: 1g

ENCHILADA SUIZA SOUP

This delicious soup brings all of the flavors of the classic enchilada dish—minus the carbs from the tortillas. Using the prepared salsa verde lets you give it all the tomatillo flavor with zero effort!

Prep Time: 10 minutes | Cook Time: 20 minutes | Total Time: 30 minutes

2 tablespoons avocado oil

6 boneless, skinless chicken thighs, cut into 1-inch pieces

½ teaspoon kosher salt, plus more for seasoning

1 teaspoon cumin

1 heaping teaspoon minced garlic

6 ounces cream cheese, cubed

16 ounces salsa verde (tomatillo salsa)

2 cups chicken broth

1 cup shredded Monterey jack cheese

Diced avocado and fresh cilantro, for garnish, optional

1. Heat the avocado oil in a large-sized heavy-bottomed pot over medium-high heat. Add the chicken thighs and season with salt, cumin, and minced garlic. Sauté the chicken until it is cooked through, about 8 minutes.

2. Reduce the heat to medium and stir in the cream cheese. Continue to stir until the cream cheese is melted, about 3 minutes. Stir in the salsa verde and the chicken broth and let simmer for 5 minutes to thicken. Season with salt to taste.

3. Serve in bowls topped with the Monterey jack cheese. Top with diced avocado and fresh cilantro if desired.

Makes 4 servings; 1¼ cups per serving | Per serving, without optional avocado: Calories: 476, Fat: 41g, Protein: 27g, Total CARBS: 3g, Fiber: 0g

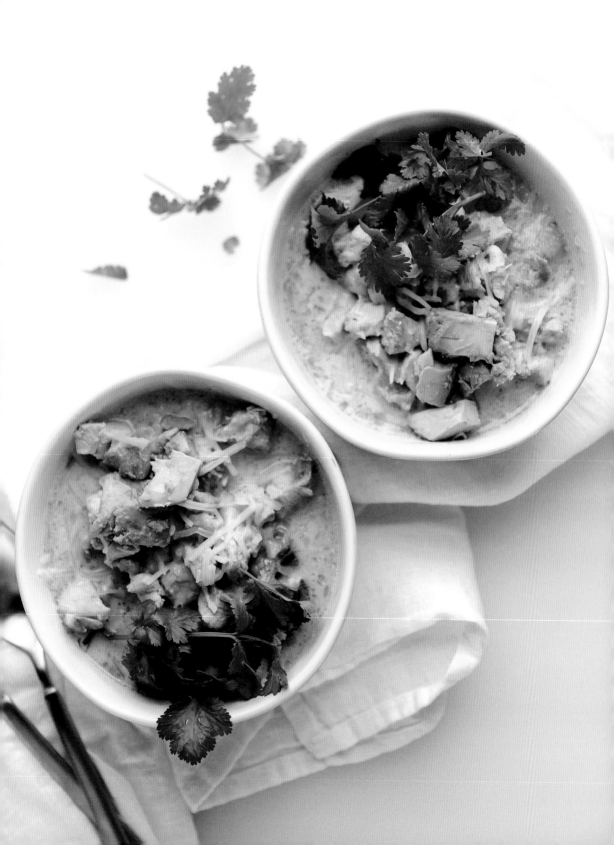

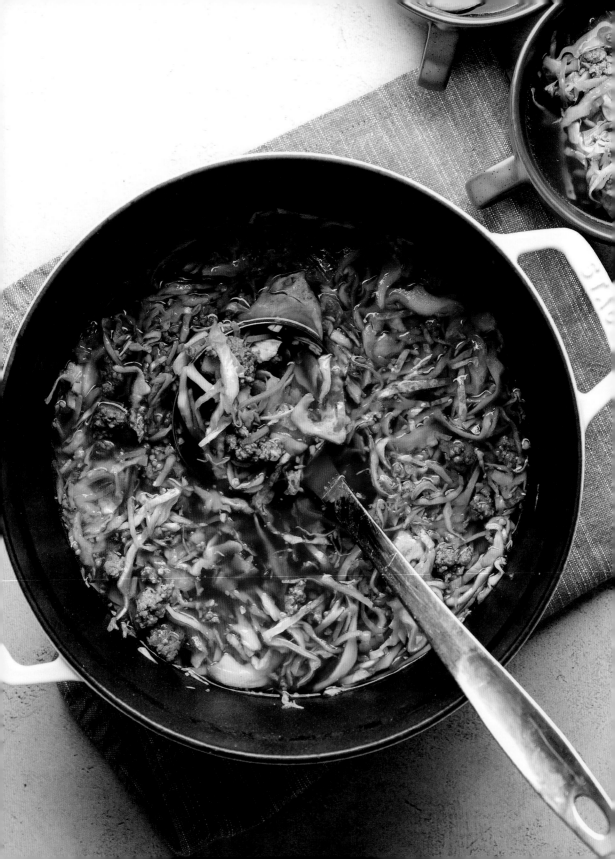

EGG ROLL SOUP

Yes, you read that right. All the delicious flavors of an egg roll, but with the ease of a quick-cooking soup—no finicky wrappers required. (As you may have guessed, creative and unconventional soup recipes are some of my favorites!) If you don't eat gluten, choose coconut aminos or tamari instead of soy sauce.

Prep Time: 5 minutes | Cook Time: 20 minutes | Total Time: 25 minutes

1 pound ground pork breakfast sausage

4 cups shredded cabbage or bagged slaw mix

2 garlic cloves, minced

2 tablespoons soy sauce, tamari, or coconut aminos

1 tablespoon rice vinegar

1 teaspoon sesame oil

4 cups chicken broth

1. In a large-sized heavy-bottomed pot over medium-high heat, cook the sausage, breaking it up with a wooden spoon, until browned and cooked through, about 8 minutes. Add the cabbage, garlic, soy sauce, rice vinegar, and sesame oil. Continue to sauté until the cabbage is wilted, about 5 minutes.

2. Stir in the chicken broth and reduce the heat to medium. Simmer for 5 minutes.

Makes 4 servings; 1¾ cups per serving | Per serving: Calories: 543, Fat: 41g, Protein: 31g, Total CARBS: 6g, Fiber: 2g

PORK AND SHRIMP MEATBALL SOUP WITH BOK CHOY

The pork and shrimp meatballs pack a savory punch in this East Asian–inspired soup—and it's extra satisfying at 2 cups per serving. Mushroom seasoning may be a new ingredient to you! It's available at many large grocery stores in the spice section. If you don't eat gluten, choose coconut aminos or tamari instead of soy sauce, and opt for a gluten-free brand of fish sauce.

Prep Time: 10 minutes | Cook Time: 40 minutes | Total Time: 50 minutes

Meatballs

1 pound ground pork

½ pound raw shrimp (any size), peeled, deveined, and finely minced

¼ cup finely chopped cilantro

2 scallions, finely chopped

1 tablespoon mushroom seasoning

1 teaspoon minced garlic

½ teaspoon kosher salt

¼ teaspoon black pepper

1 tablespoon soy sauce, tamari, or coconut aminos

½ teaspoon fish sauce

¼ teaspoon sesame oil

2 tablespoons avocado oil, divided

Soup

6 cups beef broth

3 tablespoons brown sugar sweetener

2 tablespoons soy sauce, tamari, or coconut aminos

1 tablespoon finely minced ginger

2 garlic cloves, minced

2 teaspoons sesame oil

¼ teaspoon cayenne pepper

4 baby bok choy, chopped

½ cup shredded carrots

Sliced green onions, for garnish (optional)

1. In a large mixing bowl combine all of the meatball ingredients except for the avocado oil. Stir until well mixed. Scoop the mixture, about 2 tablespoons at a time, roll into a ball, and place on a large plate or sheet tray. Repeat with the remaining mixture. You should end up with about 18 meatballs.

2. Heat 1 tablespoon of the avocado oil in a large-sized heavy-bottomed pot over medium heat. Add half of the meatballs to the pot and sear on all sides until a crust forms, about 5 minutes. Remove from the pot and set aside. Repeat with the remaining avocado oil and the other half of the meatballs. Remove from the pan and set aside.

3. Pour the beef broth into the pot and use a wooden spoon to scrape any browned bits from the bottom. Stir in the sweetener, soy sauce, ginger, garlic, sesame oil, and cayenne pepper. Add your meatballs back to the pan along with the bok choy and carrots. Cover with a lid and let simmer for 20 minutes, until the meatballs are fully cooked. Serve garnished with sliced green onions if you wish.

Makes 6 servings; 2 cups per serving | Per serving: Calories: 418, Fat: 7g, Protein: 29g, Total CARBS: 6g, Fiber: 3g

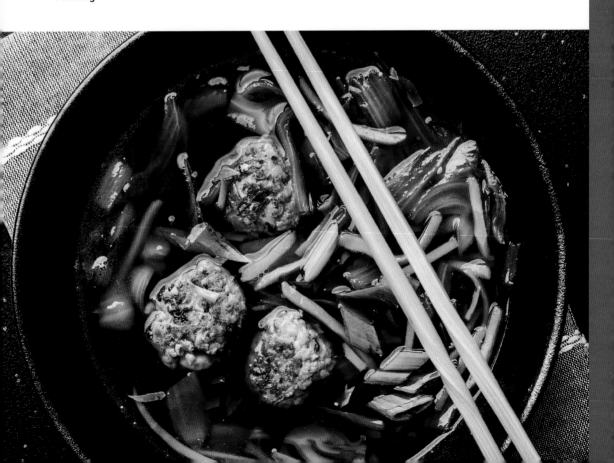

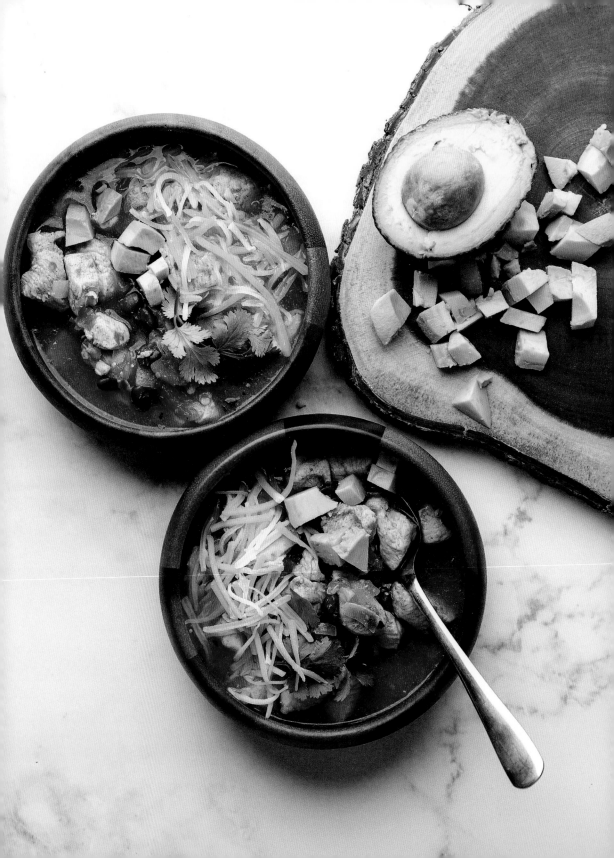

CHICKEN TACO SOUP

Do not be alarmed, but there are beans in this soup! Black soybeans give us that flavor we are so accustomed to in a taco soup or chili, with minimal carbs added. I call that a win! Look for Eden Foods brand black soybeans at your grocery store or source them online. This super flavorful and hearty soup whips up quickly so it is perfect for busy weeknights.

Prep Time: 10 minutes | Cook Time: 25 minutes | Total Time: 35 minutes

2 tablespoons avocado oil

1 small onion, diced

4 cups cooked and shredded chicken breast

1 teaspoon kosher salt

1½ teaspoons cumin

½ teaspoon garlic powder

½ teaspoon chili powder

½ teaspoon smoked paprika

2 cups chicken broth

1 (15-ounce) can black soybeans

1 (15-ounce) can diced fire-roasted tomatoes

16 ounces mild salsa verde (tomatillo salsa)

Diced avocado, for garnish (optional)

Shredded cheddar, for garnish (optional)

1. Heat the avocado oil in a large-sized heavy-bottomed pot or Dutch oven over medium heat. Add the onion and sauté until translucent, about 8 minutes. Stir in the chicken and seasonings, followed by the chicken broth, soybeans, tomatoes, and salsa verde. Give a big stir and let simmer, covered, for 15 minutes, stirring occasionally.

2. Serve topped with avocado and cheddar cheese garnish if desired.

Makes 6 servings; 1 cup per serving | Per serving (without optional avocado and cheese): Calories: 329, Fat: 17g, Total CARBS: 13g, Fiber: 5g, Protein: 43g

BACON AND MUSHROOM BEEF STEW

Everyone needs an amazing beef stew recipe in their back pocket, and I think this is the one! The addition of bacon really adds to the flavor without adding a lot of time or effort.

Prep Time: 10 minutes | Cook Time: 4 hours | Total Time: 4 hours, 10 minutes

4 slices thick-cut bacon, diced

3 pounds beef stew meat, cut into 1-inch chunks

1 teaspoon kosher salt

½ teaspoon black pepper

1 small onion, diced

3 carrots, peeled and diced

8 ounces baby bella mushrooms, quartered

½ teaspoon dried thyme

3 cups beef broth

1 teaspoon xanthan gum

1. Cook the bacon in a large-sized heavy-bottomed pot or Dutch oven over medium heat until crispy, about 8 minutes. Remove from the pot with a slotted spoon to a paper towel–lined plate and set aside. Turn the heat up to medium-high and add the beef stew meat to the remaining bacon fat in the pan. Season with salt and pepper and cook until a brown crust forms on the meat, about 5 minutes.

2. Stir in the onion, carrots, mushrooms, thyme, and beef broth. Bring to a boil, then reduce to simmer, place a lid on the pot, and cook covered for 4 hours or until the meat shreds easily with a fork.

3. Stir in the xanthan gum and bring to a boil for a few minutes, or until the stew thickens. Remove from the heat. Serve topped with the crispy bacon.

Makes 4 servings; 1 cup per serving | Per serving: Calories: 619, Fat: 27g, Total CARBS: 11g, Fiber: 4g, Protein: 79g

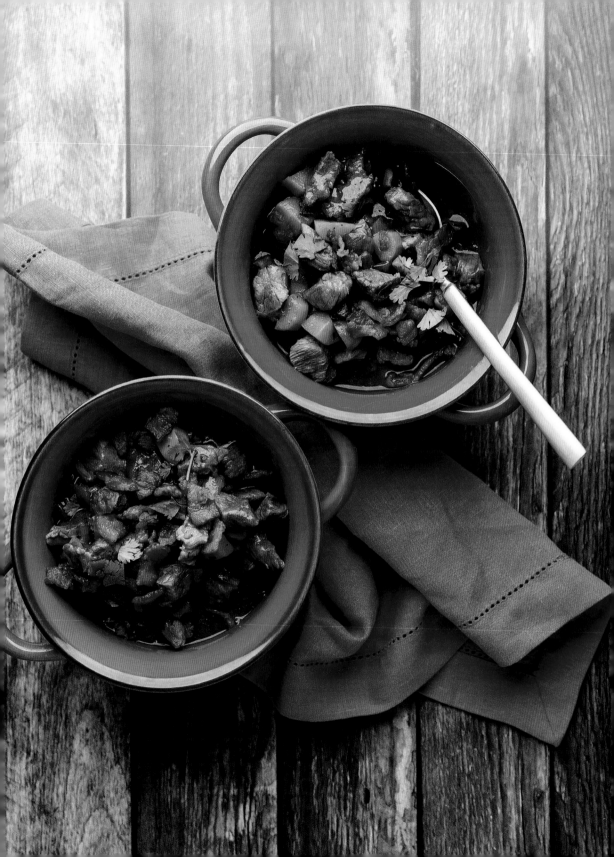

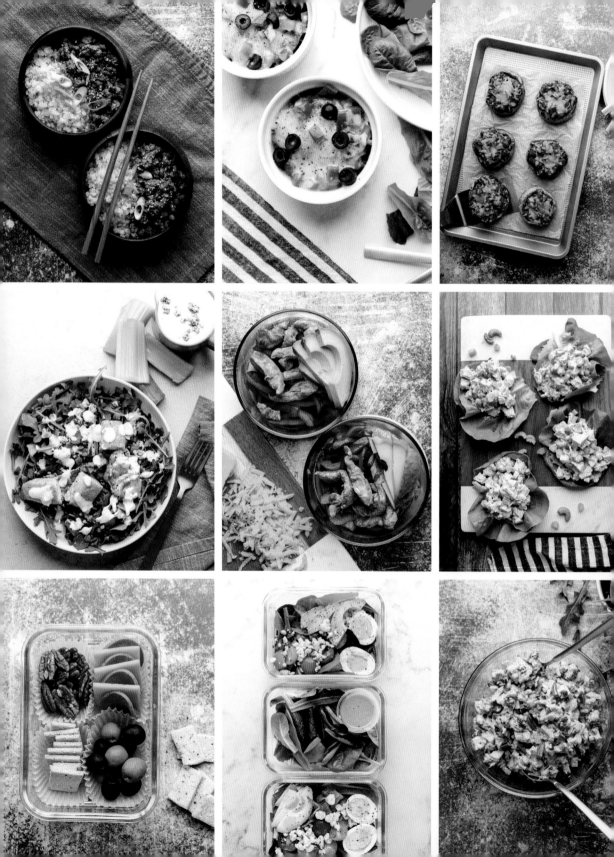

LUNCH AND MEAL PREP

BANG BANG CHICKEN AND GREEN BEANS MEAL PREP

Knock out four meals in under 30 minutes! A restaurant favorite, bang bang chicken is usually breaded and fried. This healthier stovetop version skips the breading but keeps the irresistible sweet and spicy mayo-based sauce—and it will also keep *you* satisfied for hours. If you avoid gluten, use coconut aminos or tamari instead of soy sauce. Ginger paste is a great ingredient to use in place of fresh ginger as a quick shortcut. You can usually find it in the produce section of the grocery store.

Prep Time: 10 minutes | Cook Time: 16 minutes | Total Time: 26 minutes

2 tablespoons avocado oil

6 boneless, skinless chicken thighs, cut into bite-sized pieces

½ cup mayonnaise

2 tablespoons granulated sweetener

2 tablespoons rice vinegar

2 tablespoons soy sauce, tamari, or coconut aminos

Juice of 1 lime

1 tablespoon sriracha

1 tablespoon ginger paste

1 teaspoon garlic powder

1 pound green beans, trimmed

Salt to taste

Makes 4 servings | Per serving:
Calories: 474, Fat: 37g, Total
CARBS: 13g, Fiber: 4g, Protein:
26g

1. Heat the avocado oil in a large skillet over medium-high heat. Cook the chicken thighs, stirring occasionally, for 8 minutes, until browned and cooked through. Reduce the heat to medium-low and add the remaining ingredients except the green beans and salt. Stir well and remove from the heat.

2. Set a steamer basket into a large saucepan and fill with water to a level just below the steamer. Bring to a boil. Put the beans in the steamer basket and steam for about 5 minutes or to your desired degree of tenderness (you may want to leave them on the crisper side so that they don't get too soft when reheated). Season with salt to taste.

3. Divide the chicken and the green beans evenly among 4 containers with tight-fitting lids and store in the refrigerator for up to 4 days. To reheat, microwave on high until heated through, about 1½ minutes.

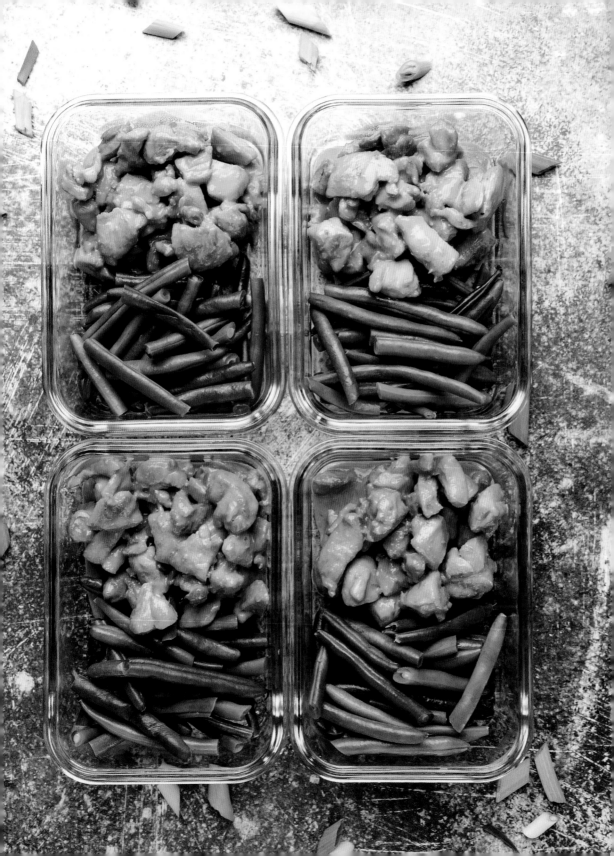

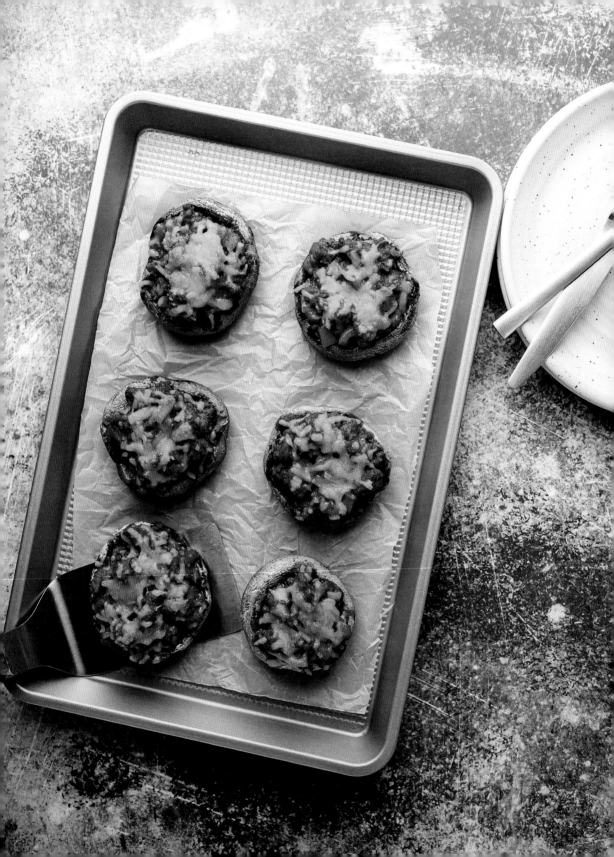

SLOPPY JOE STUFFED PORTOBELLOS

The meatiness of the portobello mushrooms really delivers as a great vehicle for sloppy joes.

Prep Time: 10 minutes | Cook Time: 10 minutes | Total Time: 20 minutes

1 pound ground beef

1 red bell pepper, diced

½ cup diced onion

½ teaspoon onion powder

½ teaspoon garlic powder

1 teaspoon kosher salt

½ teaspoon pepper

1 cup tomato sauce

2 tablespoons tomato paste

1 tablespoon apple cider vinegar

1 tablespoon Worcestershire sauce

6 medium-sized portobello mushrooms

1 cup shredded cheddar cheese

1. In a large skillet over medium-high heat, brown the ground beef, bell pepper, and onion together and season with onion powder, garlic powder, salt, and pepper. Continue to cook using a wooden spoon to break apart the meat, about 8 minutes, until the meat is cooked through and the vegetables are soft.

2. Stir in the tomato sauce, tomato paste, apple cider vinegar, and Worcestershire sauce. Cover, reduce heat to low, and let simmer for 20 minutes, stirring occasionally. Remove from the heat and set aside.

3. While the sloppy joe mixture is simmering, preheat the oven to 400°F. Use a spoon to scoop the gills and stems from the underside of the portobellos and place the mushroom caps on a baking sheet lined with parchment paper or a silicone mat. Repeat this process with each mushroom.

4. Fill each mushroom cap evenly with the sloppy joe mixture. Top evenly with shredded cheese and bake for 10 minutes until the cheese is melted.

Makes 6 servings | Per serving: Calories: 286, Fat: 18g, Total CARBS: 11g, Fiber: 4g, Protein: 22g

GINGER GARLIC PORK BOWLS MEAL PREP

I always keep frozen cauliflower rice on hand as a simple but tasty side for easy meals like this. These filling bowls are made with just five ingredients (minus the garnish!) but they're still big on flavor—and they come together in a snap, giving you four meals in under 30 minutes. Yes, please!

Prep Time: 5 minutes | Cook Time: 15 minutes | Total Time: 20 minutes

1 tablespoon avocado oil

1 pound ground pork

1 tablespoon ginger paste

1 tablespoon soy sauce, tamari, or coconut aminos

12 ounces frozen cauliflower rice, cooked according to package directions

Sliced green onion and sesame seeds for garnish (optional)

1. Heat the oil in a large skillet over medium-high heat. Add the pork and cook and crumble until browned and cooked through, about 8 minutes. Stir in the ginger and soy sauce. Remove from the heat.

2. Spoon the pork and cooked cauliflower rice equally into 4 bowl containers with airtight fitting lids. Serve topped with sliced green onion and sesame seeds for garnish if desired. Store in the refrigerator for up to 4 days. To reheat, microwave on high until heated through, about 1½ minutes.

Makes 4 servings | Per serving: Calories: 437, Fat: 36g, Total CARBS: 4g, Fiber: 2g, Protein: 22g

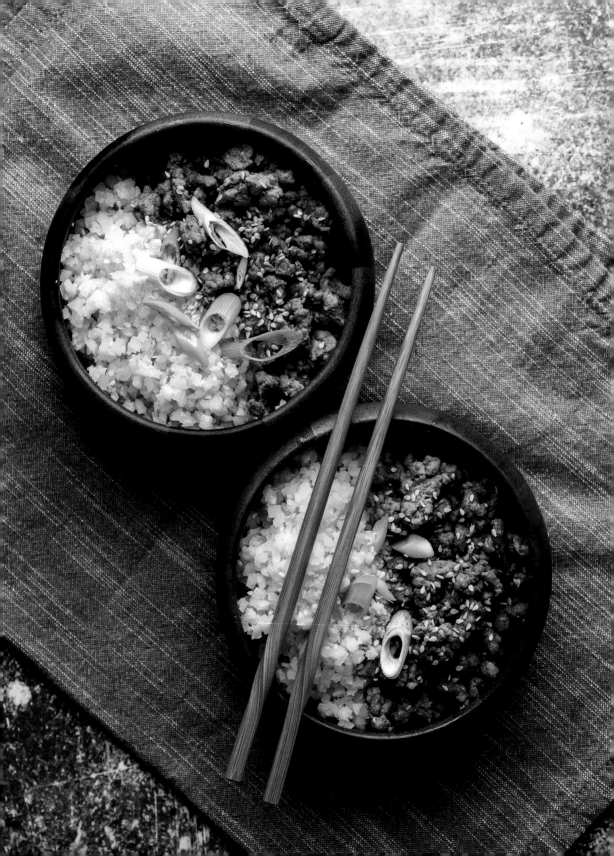

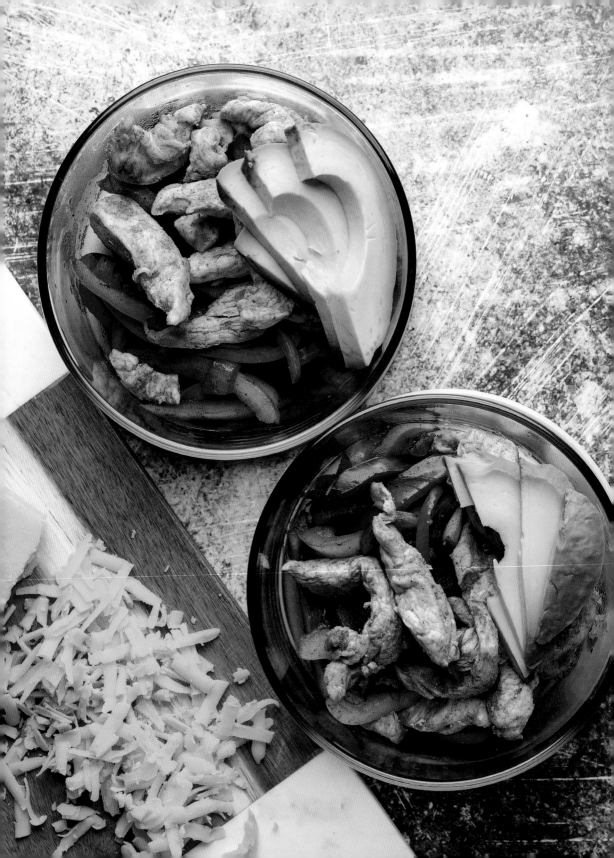

CHICKEN FAJITA BOWLS MEAL PREP

Tortillas are not required to enjoy that classic fajita flavor, but if you are feeling like you need a tortilla, there are low-carb options available or you can opt for lettuce wraps!

Prep Time: 10 minutes | Cook Time: 20 minutes | Total Time: 30 minutes

1½ teaspoons kosher salt

1½ teaspoons cumin

½ teaspoon garlic powder

½ teaspoon chili powder

½ teaspoon smoked paprika

2 tablespoons avocado oil

1½ pounds chicken breast, cut into strips

1 red bell pepper, sliced

1 yellow bell pepper, sliced

1 green bell pepper, sliced

1 white onion, sliced thin

2 tablespoons water

1 cup shredded cheddar cheese

2 avocados, peeled and sliced

1. In a small mixing bowl combine the salt, cumin, garlic powder, chili powder, and smoked paprika. Set aside.

2. Heat the oil in a large-sized heavy-bottomed skillet over medium-high heat. Add your strips of chicken breast and half of your spice mixture. Sauté the chicken for 5 minutes, until browned and cooked through. Remove from the skillet to a plate and set aside.

3. Combine the bell peppers and onion in the skillet with the remaining seasoning and 2 tablespoons of water. Cook until the vegetables are softened, about 5 minutes. Remove from the heat.

4. Divide the vegetables evenly among 4 containers with airtight lids. Place the chicken evenly on top, followed by the shredded cheese. Save the avocado and cut it right before serving. To reheat, microwave on high for 1½ minutes or until heated through, then top with the fresh avocado.

Makes 4 servings | Per serving: Calories: 457, Fat: 28g, Total CARBS: 16g, Fiber: 7g, Protein: 45g

CASHEW CHICKEN SALAD

Oh, this chicken salad may look simple, but the cashews make it extra special! I crave this chicken salad and I especially love it in butter lettuce wraps.

Prep Time: 10 minutes | Total Time: 10 minutes

12 ounces cooked chicken breast, diced

½ cup mayonnaise

1 tablespoon rice vinegar

½ cup shredded carrot

½ cup chopped celery

½ cup salted cashews

½ tablespoon granulated sweetener

Salt and pepper to taste

Combine all ingredients in a large mixing bowl and mix well. Season with salt and pepper to taste.

Makes 4 servings; ¾ cup per serving | Per serving: Calories: 389, Fat: 28g, Total CARBS: 7g, Fiber: 1g, Protein: 27g

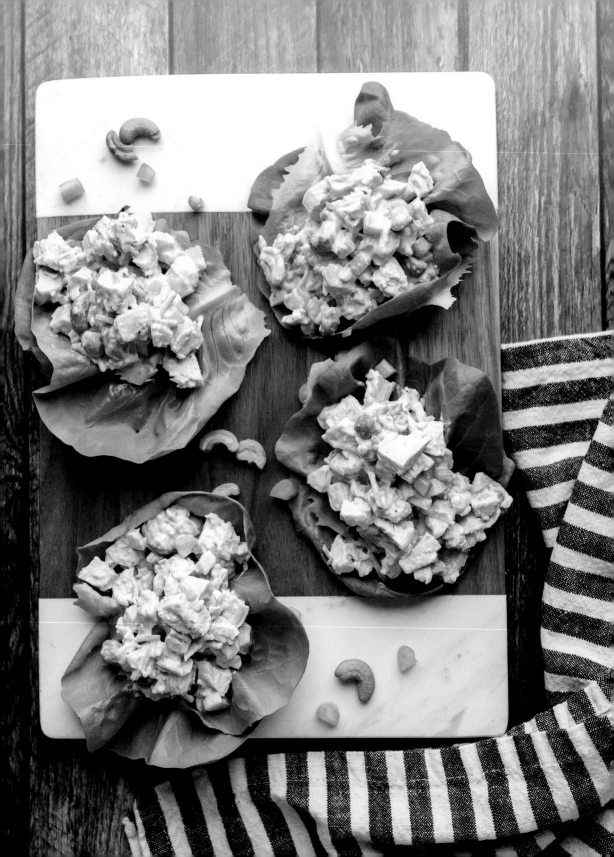

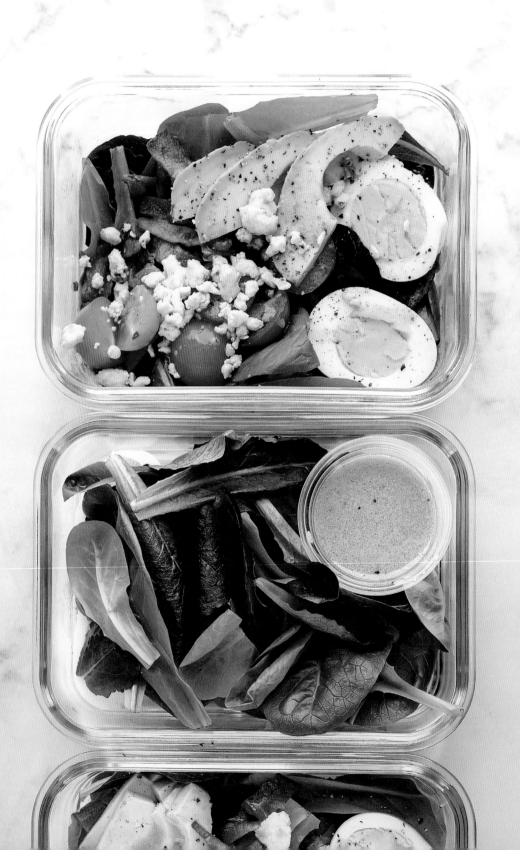

COBB SALAD MEAL PREP

Yes, you can meal prep salads! The trick is to find a salad green that stands up to prepping such as arugula or romaine. Keep your dressing separate until you are ready to eat. I often keep cooked bacon on hand so I have it ready for salads like this one and My Favorite Salmon Salad Meal Prep on page 116. To whip up a batch, see my easy method—Oven-Cooked Bacon—on page 263.

Prep Time: 10 minutes | Cook Time: 20 minutes | Total Time: 30 minutes

4 large eggs

8 slices thick bacon, cooked and crumbled

4 ounces crumbled blue cheese

16 cherry tomatoes, halved

8 cups sturdy salad greens such as arugula or romaine

2 avocados, sliced (cut right before serving)

Dressing

3 tablespoons olive oil

3 tablespoons red wine vinegar

1 tablespoon Dijon mustard

Salt and pepper to taste

1. Place the eggs in a small saucepan and cover with water. Bring to a boil, then reduce to a simmer and cook for 10 minutes. Remove the pan from the heat and place in the sink. Run cold water over the eggs until the water in the pan is cooled. Let sit for 5 minutes, then remove the eggshells. Slice in half.

2. Divide all salad ingredients (except the avocados) among 4 containers with airtight lids, leaving the greens on top for the least amount of wilting.

3. In a small mixing bowl whisk together the dressing ingredients until fully emulsified. Divide the dressing among 4 (2-ounce) dressing containers with tight-fitting lids. Store the salads and dressing in the refrigerator for up to 4 days. Top each serving with ½ avocado, sliced, just before enjoying.

Makes 4 servings | Per serving: Calories: 518, Fat: 42g, Total CARBS: 14g, Fiber: 10g, Protein: 20g

PIZZA BOWLS MEAL PREP

All the flavors of pizza with none of the carbs, a satisfying pizza bowl is perfect for a meal prep lunch for you, or to feed some picky, hungry kiddos a quick dinner. Get creative with other low-carb pizza toppings you love—you might try it with mushrooms, bacon, zucchini, broccoli, or hot peppers.

Prep Time: 15 minutes | Cook Time: 10 minutes | Total Time: 25 minutes

1 pound breakfast sausage

¾ cup marinara sauce (I like Rao's)

2 cups shredded mozzarella cheese

48 pepperoni slices

¾ cup diced bell pepper

2 ounces black olives

1. Cook and crumble the sausage in a large skillet over medium-high heat until cooked through, about 8 minutes. Drain on a paper towel–lined plate and set aside.

2. Gather 6 microwave safe meal prep bowls with tight-fitting lids. Divide the cooked crumbled sausage among the bowls. Top each with 2 tablespoons marinara sauce, ⅓ cup mozzarella cheese, 8 pepperoni slices, 1 tablespoon diced bell pepper, and 1 tablespoon olives. Cover with the lids and store in the refrigerator for up to 1 week.

3. To heat, remove the lid from the bowl and microwave on high in 1-minute increments until heated through and the cheese is melted.

Makes 6 servings | Per serving: Calories: 456, Fat: 36g, Total CARBS: 4g, Fiber: 1g, Protein: 29g

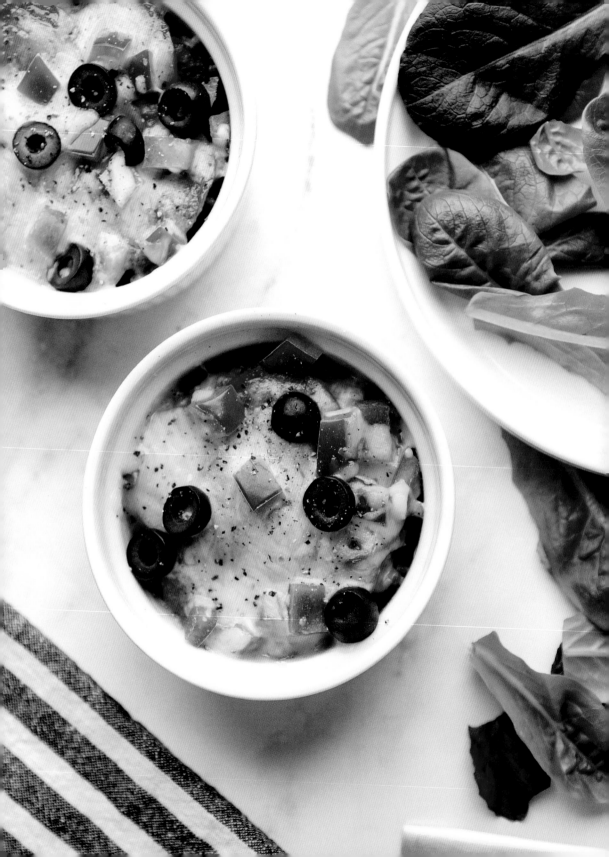

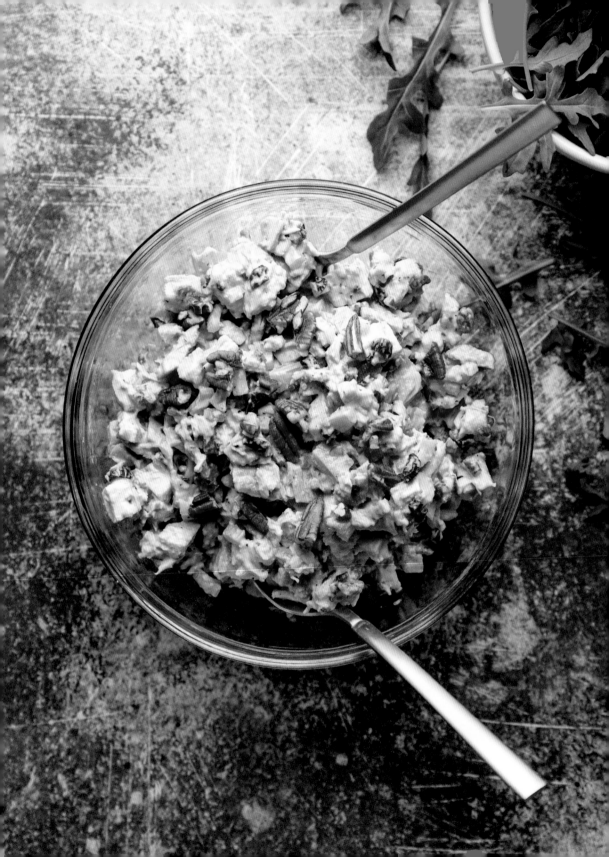

"HONEY" DIJON CHICKEN SALAD

With Homemade "Honey" Mustard Sauce

Enjoy this delightful chicken salad as is, in a low-carb tortilla, or in lettuce cups.
To save time, you don't even need to mix the sauce separately—you can simply
combine all the ingredients for salad and sauce in a large mixing bowl and toss
to combine! The "honey" mustard sauce can also be used as a salad dressing or a
dipping sauce that's just perfect for chicken tenders. Yum!

Prep Time: 10 minutes | Cook Time: 15 minutes | Total Time: 25 minutes

"Honey" Mustard Sauce

2 tablespoons powdered
   sweetener

1 teaspoon garlic powder

½ teaspoon kosher salt

¼ teaspoon pepper

½ cup mayonnaise

1 tablespoon apple cider
   vinegar

1 tablespoon yellow mustard

1 tablespoon Dijon mustard

Chicken Salad

12 ounces chicken breast,
   cooked and diced

½ cup chopped pecans

½ cup chopped celery

¼ cup chopped dried
   unsweetened cranberries

1. Combine all the sauce ingredients in a large
   mixing bowl and stir well.

2. Add the chicken, pecans, celery, and cranberries
   and toss to evenly coat them in the sauce.

Makes 4 servings; 1 cup per serving | Per serving: Calories: 422, Fat: 29g, Total CARBS: 9g, Fiber: 1g,

Protein: 27g

MY FAVORITE SALMON SALAD MEAL PREP

This is the salad I lived on for months during my weight loss journey. I could seriously eat it every day and never get tired of it—so that's why I like to meal prep four servings at a time! The salmon and bacon bring plenty of richness to make this salad feel like a satisfying meal. My Lightened-Up Blue Cheese Dressing (page 261) is on the lighter side to balance it out.

Prep Time: 10 minutes | Cook Time: 10 minutes | Total Time: 20 minutes

4 (4-ounce) boneless salmon planks

½ teaspoon kosher salt

½ teaspoon garlic powder

8 cups arugula

4 slices thick bacon, cooked and crumbled

4 ounces crumbled blue cheese

Salt and pepper to taste

8 tablespoons Lightened-Up Blue Cheese Dressing (page 261)

1. Line a sheet pan with foil and spray with cooking spray. Preheat the oven to high broil.

2. Place the salmon on the sheet tray and season with salt and garlic powder. Broil the salmon for 8 minutes, until the internal temperature registers 125°F using a meat thermometer.

3. Gather 4 meal prep bowls with tight-fitting lids. Layer the bowls with the arugula, salmon, bacon, blue cheese, and season with salt and pepper to taste. Divide the dressing evenly among 4 (2-ounce) dressing cups with lids. Place the lids on the salad bowls and store in the refrigerator for up to 4 days.

Makes 4 servings | Per serving: Calories: 344, Fat: 23g, Total CARBS: 8g, Fiber: 1g, Protein: 27g

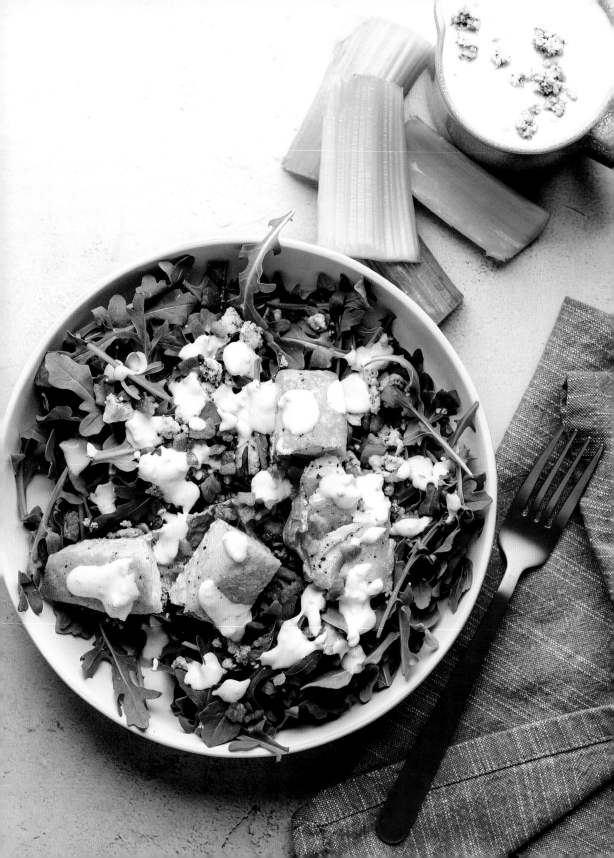

SNACK BOXES WITH HOMEMADE BLACK PEPPER CRACKERS

Who didn't love those cheese and cracker boxes as a kid? I know I did! This adult version will bring back memories but will also nourish you with the hearty cheese, salami, pecans, olives, and delicious homemade black pepper crackers. The cracker recipe easily doubles so you can have extra for snacking!

Prep Time: 15 minutes | Cook Time: 20 minutes | Total Time: 35 minutes

Black Pepper Crackers

1 cup almond flour (plus a little more for dusting)

¼ teaspoon garlic powder

1 large egg, beaten

¼ teaspoon sea salt

Freshly cracked black pepper

Snack Boxes

112g (1 cup) sliced cheddar cheese

112g (1 cup) sliced Genoa salami

80g (¾ cup) Castelvetrano olives

80g (¾ cup) black olives

112g (1 cup) shelled pecans

1. To make the crackers: Preheat the oven to 300°F and line a sheet tray with parchment paper.

2. Combine the almond flour and garlic powder in a large mixing bowl. Stir in the egg and mix well until a dough forms.

3. Turn the dough out onto an almond-floured work surface and use a rolling pin to roll the dough into a large rectangle ⅛ of an inch thick. Season with the sea salt and black pepper. Use a pizza cutter or sharp knife to cut the dough into approximately 40 (1 × 2–inch) crackers. Remove the crackers with a thin metal spatula and place on the prepared baking sheet.

4. Bake for 20 minutes or until they are lightly browned around the edges. Cool completely, then store in an airtight container.

5. To assemble each snack box: insert 4 cupcake liners into a 6 × 5–inch meal prep container with a tight-fitting lid. In one muffin liner,

place 28g of cheese and 28g of salami. In the second liner, place 20g of each kind of olive; in the third liner, place 28g pecans; and in the last liner, nest 5 homemade crackers. (Assemble the day of consuming as the crackers will become soft if left to sit too long in the refrigerator.)

Makes 40 crackers (5 crackers per serving) and 4 snack boxes | Per serving: Calories: 622, Fat: 57g, Total CARBS: 10g, Fiber: 6g, Protein: 24g

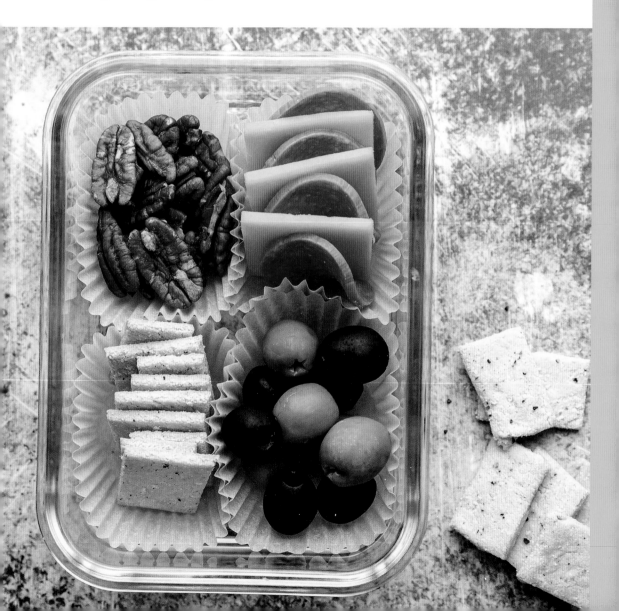

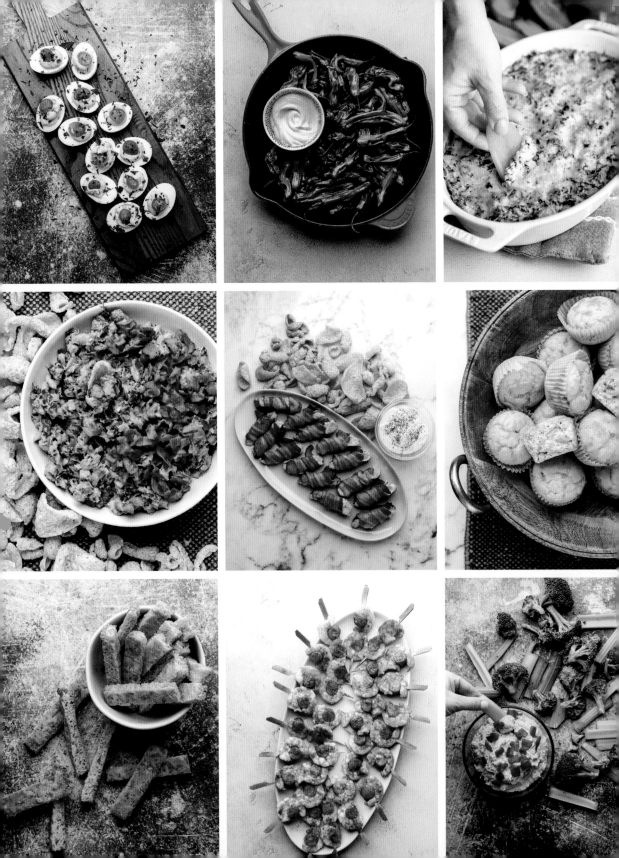

APPETIZERS AND SNACKS

LOADED GUACAMOLE

This classic appetizer is made even more delicious with crispy bacon. Everything's better with bacon! Serve with cut fresh veggies or pork rinds for the perfect keto-friendly treat.

Prep Time: 10 minutes | Cook Time: 15 minutes | Total Time: 25 minutes

½ pound bacon, diced

4 medium avocados, peeled, seeds removed, and diced

2 Roma tomatoes, diced

1 cup chopped cilantro

¾ cup diced red onion

Juice of 1 lime

1½ teaspoons garlic powder

½ teaspoon kosher salt

1. Heat a large skillet over medium-high heat. Sauté the bacon until crispy, 10–15 minutes. Remove from the pan with a slotted spoon and transfer to a plate lined with paper towels to drain and cool slightly. Set aside.

2. In a large mixing bowl combine the rest of the ingredients and half of the bacon. Stir gently to combine. Top with the remaining bacon and serve immediately.

Makes approximately 4 cups, 8 servings (½ cup per serving) | Per serving: Calories: 230, Fat: 17g, Total CARBS: 8g, Fiber: 6g, Protein: 12g

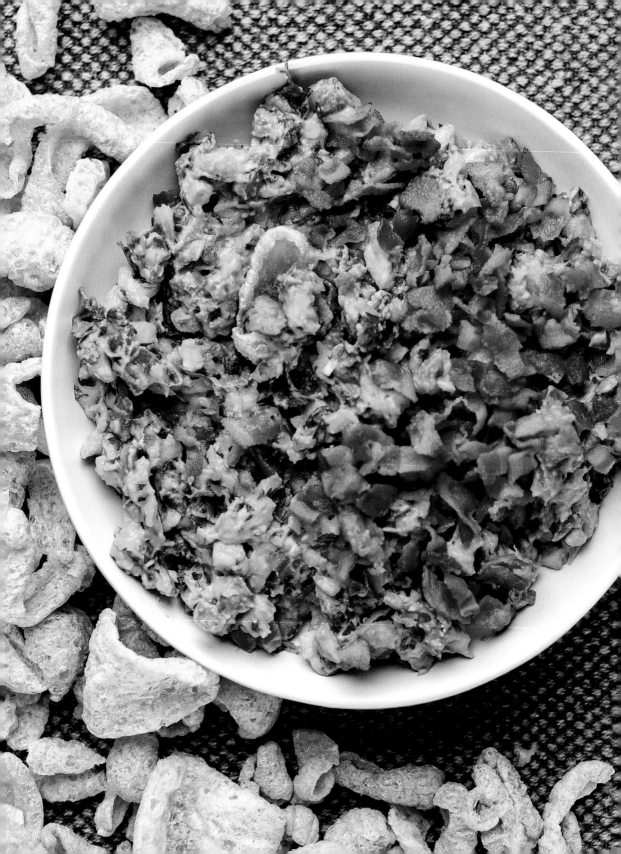

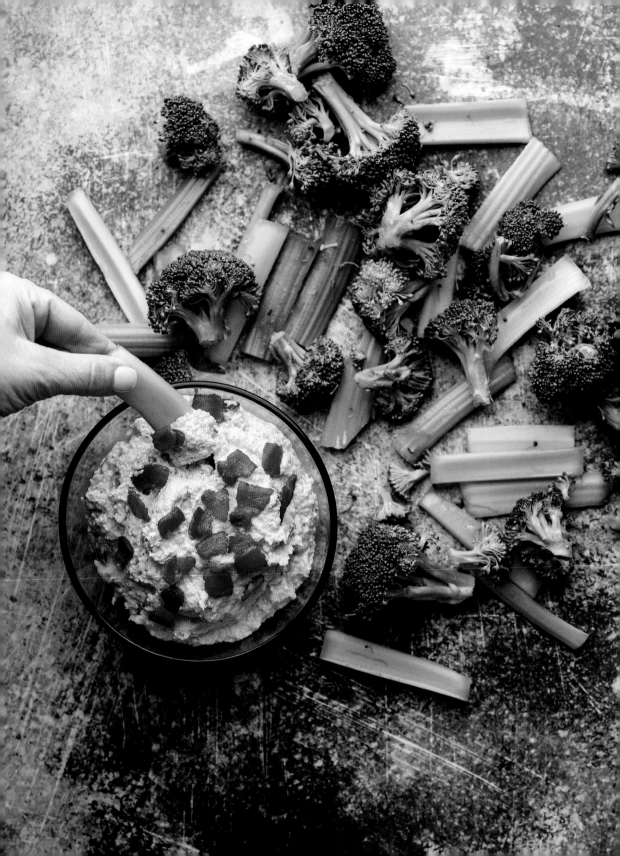

BACON, CHEDDAR, AND CAULIFLOWER DIP

Don't tell anyone there's cauliflower in this delicious dip because they will never know! What a great way to get in some extra veggies! Serve with fresh-cut veggies (I especially like broccoli and celery with this dip) or pork rinds.

Prep Time: 10 minutes | Cook Time: 15 minutes | Total Time: 25 minutes

½ pound bacon, diced

12 ounces frozen cauliflower rice, prepared according to package directions

1½ cups shredded cheddar cheese

4 ounces cream cheese, softened

1 tablespoon dried chives

1 garlic clove, minced

½ teaspoon garlic powder

½ teaspoon kosher salt

¼ teaspoon pepper

1. Heat a large skillet over medium-high heat and sauté the bacon until crispy, 10–15 minutes. Remove from the pan with a slotted spoon to a plate lined with paper towels and set aside.

2. Combine all of the ingredients except the crispy bacon in a food processor and blend until smooth. Scrape the dip from the food processor to a mixing bowl and fold in most of the crispy bacon. Top the dip with the remaining bacon pieces just before serving.

Makes 2½ cups dip, 8 servings (⅓ cup per serving) | Per serving: Calories: 243, Fat: 18g, Total CARBS: 3g, Fiber: 1g, Protein: 16g

CHEESY "CORNBREAD" MUFFINS

These cornbread-style muffins (made without corn!) taste remarkably like those traditional ones your grandma used to make, only with much fewer carbs and no sugar!

Prep Time: 5 minutes | Cook Time: 20 minutes | Total Time: 25 minutes

2 cups almond flour

1 cup shredded cheddar cheese

¼ cup granulated sweetener

½ teaspoon kosher salt

½ teaspoon baking powder

4 large eggs, beaten

1 cup half-and-half

¼ cup butter, melted and cooled slightly

1. Preheat the oven to 350°F and line a 12-cup muffin tin with liners. Spray the inside of the liners with nonstick spray.

2. In a mixing bowl, whisk together the almond flour, cheddar cheese, sweetener, salt, and baking powder. Stir in the beaten eggs, half-and-half, and melted butter until fully combined.

3. Divide the batter evenly among the muffin cups and bake for 30 minutes or until a toothpick inserted in the center comes out clean. Let cool completely in the pan. Store any leftovers in the refrigerator in an airtight container for up to 1 week.

Makes 12 "cornbread" muffins; 1 per serving | Per serving: Calories: 232, Fat: 21g, Total CARBS: 5g, Fiber: 2g, Protein: 9g

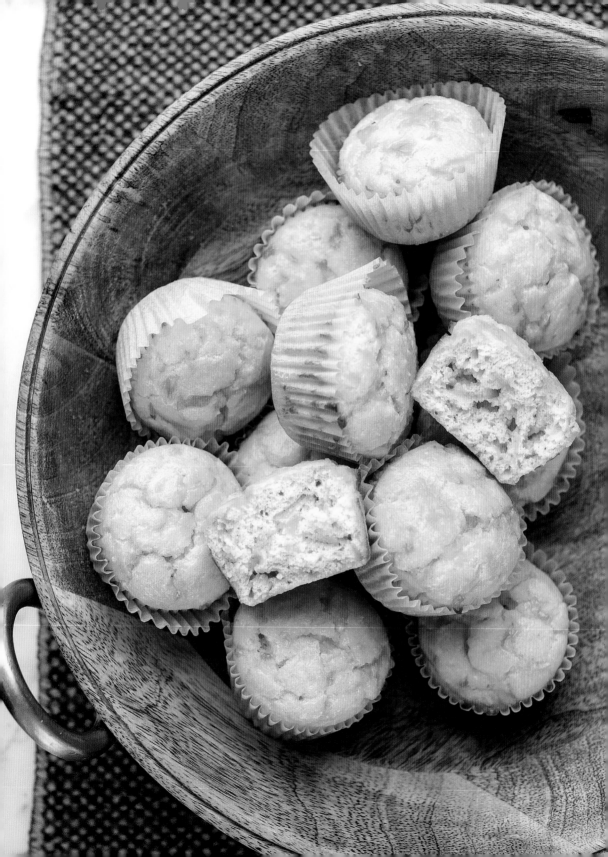

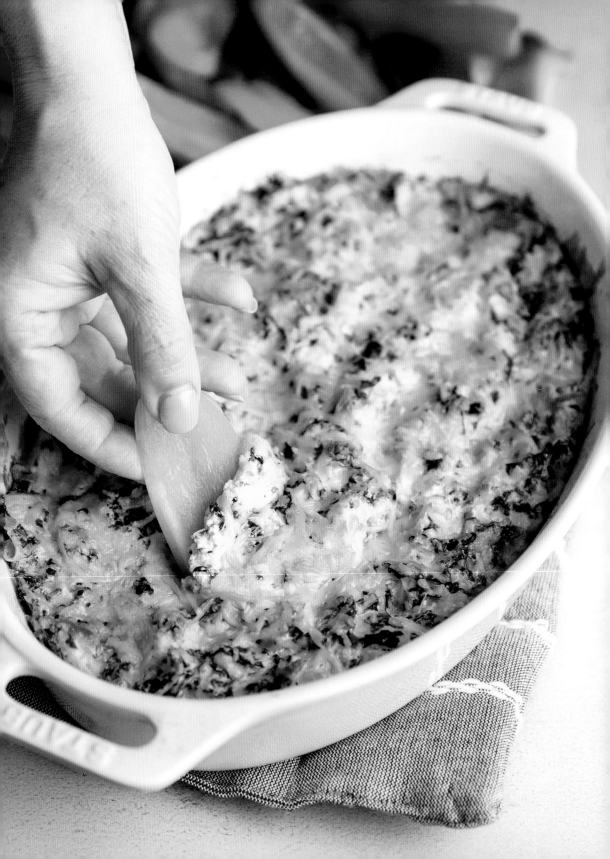

BAKED SPINACH ARTICHOKE DIP

Spinach and artichoke dip is always my favorite dip at any party or appetizer at restaurants. Baking it gives it a wonderfully cheesy, slightly crispy top layer. Serve this with vegetable sticks or pork rinds and no one will ever guess they are eating keto.

Prep Time: 10 minutes | Cook Time: 30 minutes | Total Time: 40 minutes

12 ounces frozen chopped spinach, thawed and drained

1 (13-ounce) can quartered artichoke hearts, drained and chopped

8 ounces cream cheese, softened and cut into 1-inch cubes

1 cup sour cream

1 cup shredded mozzarella cheese

1 cup Parmesan cheese, divided

4 garlic cloves, minced

1 teaspoon kosher salt

½ teaspoon black pepper

1. Preheat the oven to 400°F and grease the inside of a 3-quart baking dish.

2. Combine all of the ingredients in a large mixing bowl, except ½ cup Parmesan cheese. Mix well. Pour into the prepared baking dish and spread in an even layer. Top with the remaining Parmesan.

3. Bake for 30 minutes or until the top is golden brown. Serve immediately.

Makes 10 servings | Per serving: Calories: 212, Fat: 17g, Total CARBS: 5g, Fiber: 1g, Protein: 9g

HOMESTYLE DEVILED EGGS

The ground mustard and dill pickle relish really give a nice kick to the traditional deviled egg recipe. The sliced cherry tomatoes not only make them look pretty, but also add to the flavor!

Prep Time: 15 minutes | Cook Time: 15 minutes | Total Time: 30 minutes

6 large eggs

¼ cup mayonnaise

2 tablespoons dill pickle relish

1 teaspoon ground mustard

Sliced cherry tomatoes, for garnish

Chopped fresh parsley, for garnish (optional)

Makes 6 servings; 2 halves per serving | Per serving: Calories: 144, Fat: 12g, Total CARBS: 1g, Fiber: 0g, Protein: 7g

1. Place the eggs in a small saucepan and cover with water. Bring to a boil, then reduce to a simmer and cook for 10 minutes. Remove the pan from the heat and place in the sink. Run cold water over the eggs until the water in the pan is cooled. Let sit for 5 minutes until cool enough to handle, then remove the eggshells.

2. Using a sharp knife, cut each egg in half, lengthwise. Scoop out the yolks into a small bowl. Arrange the hard-cooked whites on a serving platter.

3. To the yolks, add the mayonnaise, pickle relish, and ground mustard. Mix with a fork, smashing the yolks, until the mixture is smooth. (Alternatively, you can use an electric mixer.)

4. Scoop the mixture evenly into the white shells with a spoon, or use a piping bag for a neater presentation.

5. Top with the sliced tomatoes and parsley if desired.

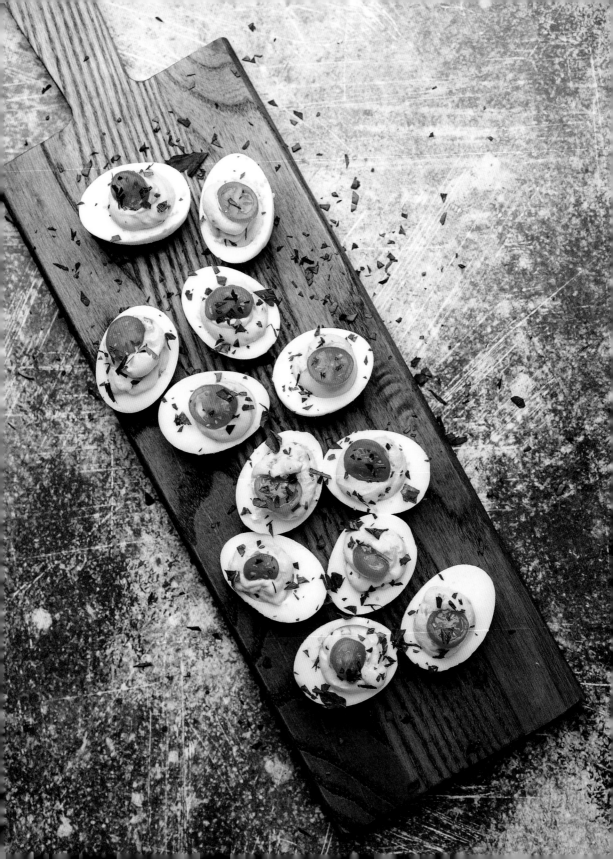

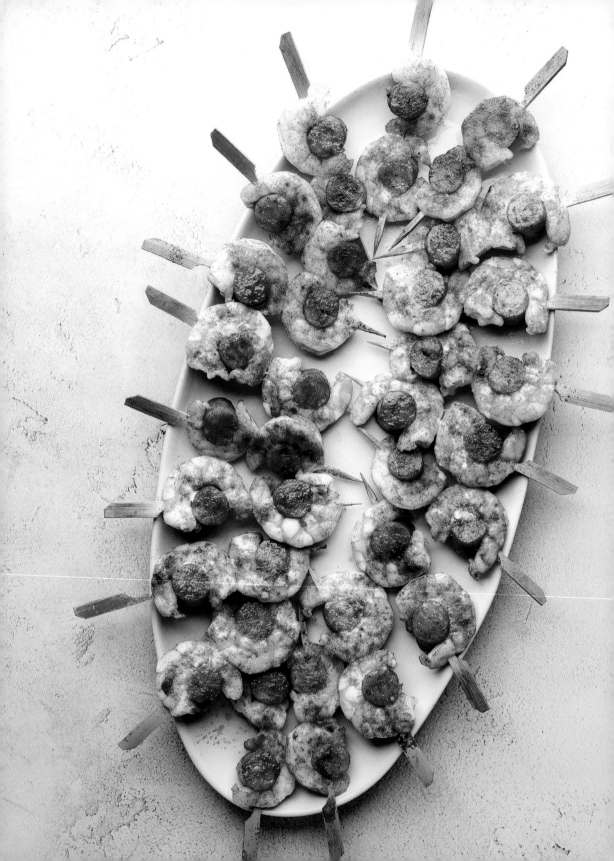

SHRIMP AND KIELBASA SKEWERS

Shrimp and smoky kielbasa make the perfect combo in this simple appetizer. These are so easy to assemble that you will likely want to make them regularly for just a weeknight dinner.

Prep Time: 10 minutes | Cook Time: 16 minutes | Total Time: 26 minutes

20 (6-inch-long) skewers

2 teaspoons smoked paprika

1 teaspoon kosher salt

¼ teaspoon garlic powder

¼ teaspoon onion powder

⅛ teaspoon cayenne pepper

8 ounces, 1-inch diameter, smoked sausage, cut into 1-inch pieces

1½ pounds large shrimp, peeled and deveined

3 tablespoons butter, melted

Makes 20 skewers; 2 skewers per serving | Per serving: Calories: 169, Fat: 10g, Total CARBS: 0g, Fiber: 0g, Protein: 19g

1. Preheat the oven to high broil. Line a rimmed baking sheet with foil. Place 20 (6-inch-long) skewers in a bowl of water to soak.

2. Mix the smoked paprika, salt, garlic powder, onion powder, and cayenne together in a small mixing bowl. Set aside.

3. Assemble your ingredients and skewers. Arrange 1 slice of sausage in the curve of 1 shrimp and push the skewer through the shrimp and sausage. Each skewer will hold 2 shrimp and sausages. Repeat the process with the remaining shrimp. Place on the lined baking sheet.

4. Season both sides of the skewers with the seasoning mixture. Place in the oven on the middle rack and broil for 6–8 minutes on each side, watching carefully so they do not burn. The shrimp will be opaque and the sausage will be sizzling.

5. Remove from the oven and use a basting brush to brush the skewers on both sides with the melted butter.

PAN BLISTERED SHISHITO PEPPERS WITH AIOLI

The tangy and spicy aioli is a perfect accompaniment to blistered shishito peppers. Most shishitos are mild, but once in a while you'll come across one that brings the heat! Feel free to increase the amount of sriracha for even more spice.

Prep Time: 5 minutes | Cook Time: 10 minutes | Total Time: 15 minutes

2 tablespoons avocado oil

12 ounces shishito peppers

½ teaspoon kosher salt

½ cup mayonnaise

½ teaspoon garlic powder

1 teaspoon sriracha

Juice of ½ lemon

1. Heat the oil in a large skillet over medium-high heat. Add the peppers and season with salt. Toss to coat in the oil. Cook, stirring occasionally, for about 10 minutes or until the peppers start to blister and brown. Remove from the heat.

2. While the peppers are cooking, in a small mixing bowl combine the mayo, garlic powder, sriracha, and lemon juice. Serve with the peppers.

Makes 4 servings | Per serving: Calories: 265, Fat: 28g, Total CARBS: 4g, Fiber: 2g, Protein: 1g

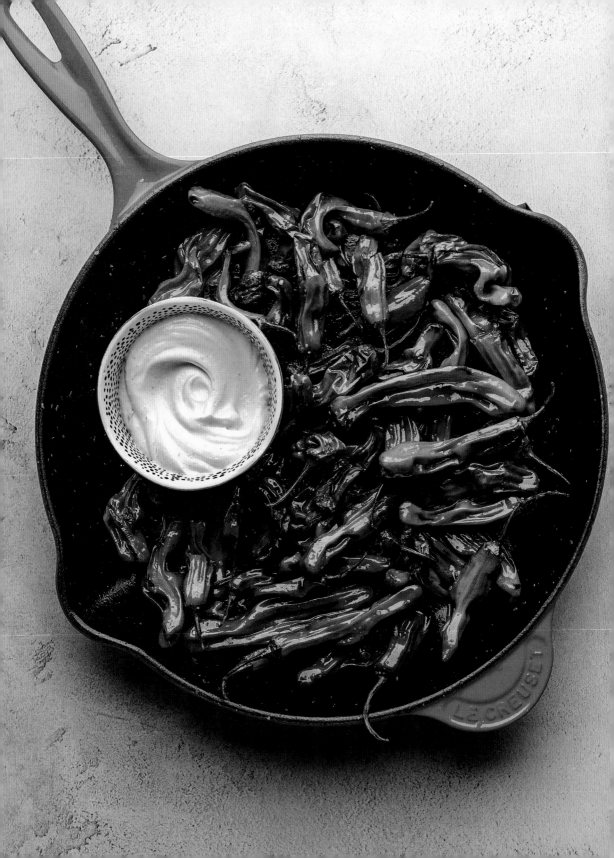

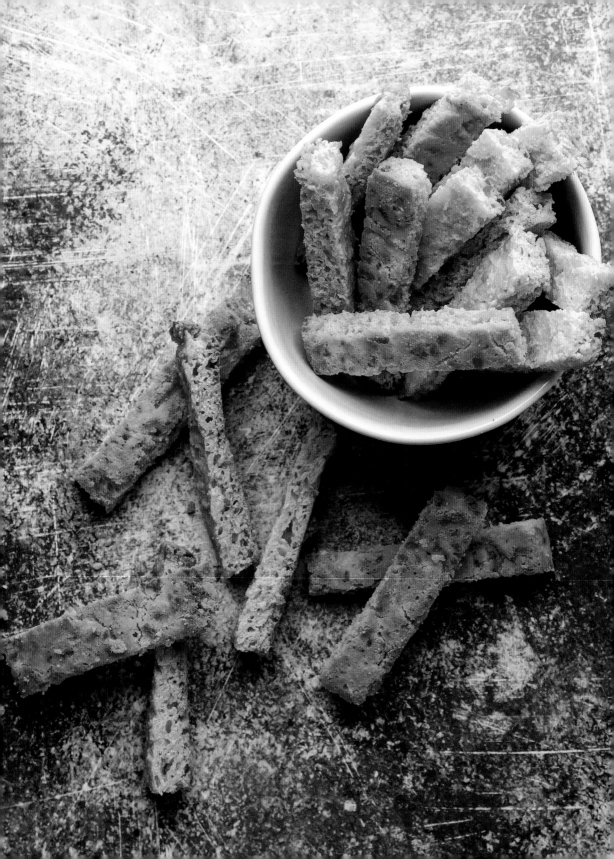

CHEESE STRAWS

Cheese straws are a fantastic handheld snack to serve at a party—I especially love to make them during the holidays. The sharpness from the cheese complements the slight spice from the cayenne.

Prep Time: 5 minutes | Cook Time: 50 minutes | Total Time: 55 minutes

2 cups almond flour

1 teaspoon garlic powder

½ teaspoon cayenne pepper

¼ teaspoon kosher salt

¼ teaspoon baking powder

3 large eggs

1 cup shredded cheddar cheese

½ cup melted butter

1. Preheat the oven to 350°F. Line the bottom of a quarter-rimmed baking sheet with parchment paper and spray with cooking spray.

2. In a large mixing bowl combine the almond flour, garlic powder, cayenne, salt, and baking powder. Add the eggs, cheese, and butter and stir until the dough is well mixed.

3. Spread the mixture evenly in the prepared baking sheet and bake for 20 minutes. Remove from the oven and let cool for 10 minutes.

4. Use a sharp knife to cut the bread lengthwise down the center of the pan, then into ½-inch strips. This will make approximately 26 cheese straws. Transfer the straws to a larger baking sheet to spread them out a bit and place back in the oven for 20 minutes, or until crispy.

Makes 26 cheese straws; 1 per serving | Per serving: Calories: 109, Fat: 10g, Total Carbs: 2g, Fiber: 1g, Protein: 4g

BACON WRAPPED PICKLE POPPERS

You may think this combination sounds crazy but trust me, these cheesy, salty snacks will be a big hit at your next party!

Prep Time: 15 minutes | Cook Time: 25 minutes | Total Time: 40 minutes

7 medium-sized dill pickles

¾ cup cream cheese, softened

¾ cup shredded cheddar cheese

1 teaspoon garlic powder

Salt and pepper to taste

14 slices thin bacon

1. Preheat the oven to 425°F and line a baking sheet with foil or parchment paper.

2. Cut each pickle in half lengthwise and scrape out the inner flesh and seeds. Place the pickle halves on the baking sheet.

3. In a medium-sized mixing bowl combine the cream cheese, cheddar cheese, and garlic powder. Season with salt and pepper to taste. Fill each pickle half evenly with the cheese mixture. Wrap each pickle half with a slice of bacon. If the bacon is too long, trim the end. Secure the bacon with toothpicks.

4. Bake for 25 minutes or until the bacon is crispy. Serve immediately.

Makes 14 pickle poppers; 2 per serving | Per serving: Calories: 227, Fat: 19g, Total CARBS: 4g, Fiber: 0g, Protein: 9g

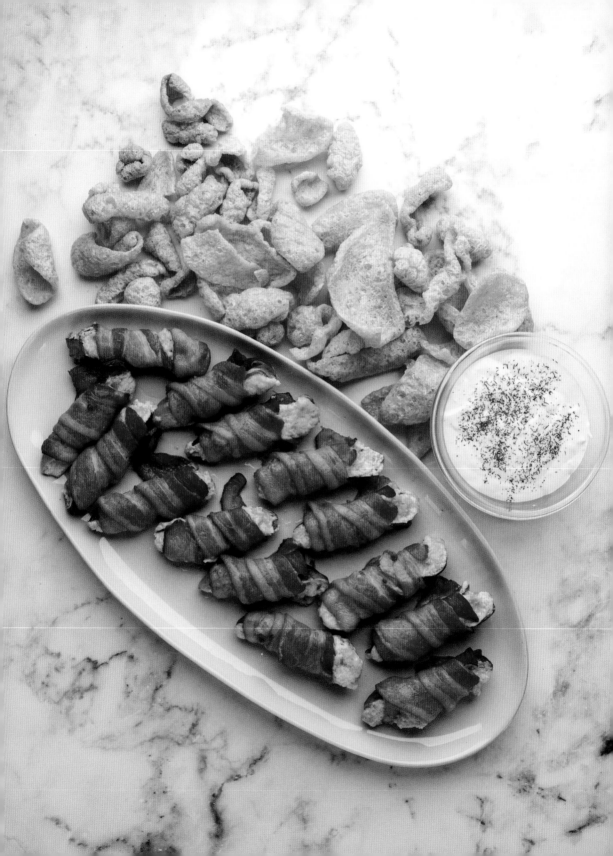

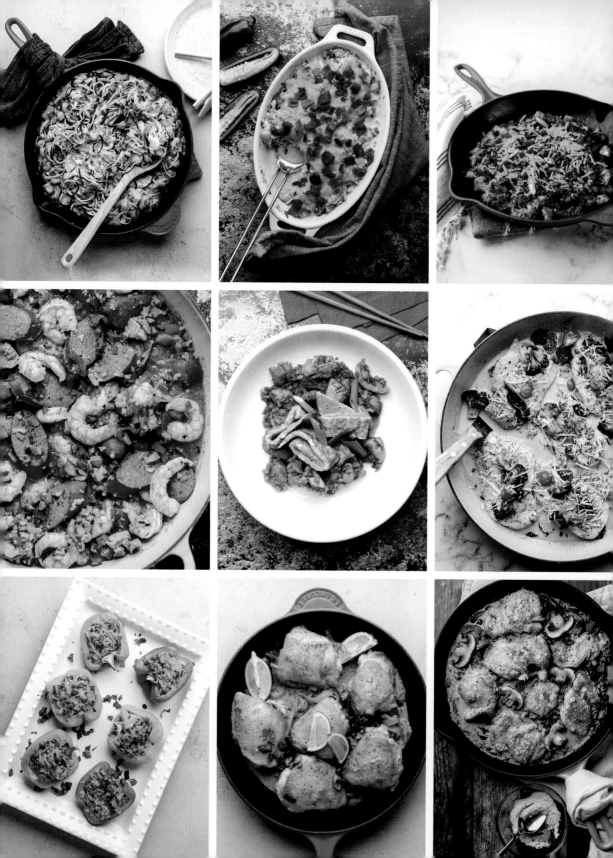

CHICKEN

SHREDDED CHICKEN BREAST

Shredded chicken breast is so versatile and the seasoning in this recipe cannot be beat. Use this chicken for meal prep or pair it with vegetables for a quick dinner.

Prep Time: 5 minutes | Cook Time: 25 minutes | Total Time: 30 minutes

1½ pounds boneless, skinless chicken breast

1 teaspoon smoked paprika

1 teaspoon garlic powder

½ teaspoon oregano

½ teaspoon onion powder

½ teaspoon kosher salt

Makes 6 servings (4 ounces per serving) | Per serving: Calories: 150, Fat: 1g, Total CARBS: 1g, Fiber: 0g, Protein: 32g

1. Preheat the oven to 400°F and grease a 9 × 13–inch baking dish with oil or cooking spray. Place the chicken in a single layer in the baking dish.

2. In a small mixing bowl combine the spices. Coat both sides of the chicken with the spice mixture.

3. Bake for 25 minutes or until the chicken has an internal temperature of 165°F. Use a meat thermometer inserted into the center of the chicken breast to test for doneness.

4. Remove from the oven and let rest for 10 minutes. Use 2 forks to shred the chicken. The chicken will release a lot of liquid while cooking, so pour any pan drippings back into the shredded chicken for moisture.

Note: Almost any time I cook chicken, I use this seasoning blend—so I like to keep a slightly larger batch premixed to make a quick chicken salad or easy meal prep. Combine 1½ teaspoons smoked paprika, 1½ teaspoons garlic powder, ¾ teaspoon oregano, ¾ teaspoon onion powder, and ¾ teaspoon kosher salt in an airtight container and store for up to 1 month. This is enough seasoning for 1 whole chicken, 8 chicken thighs, or 4 chicken breasts.

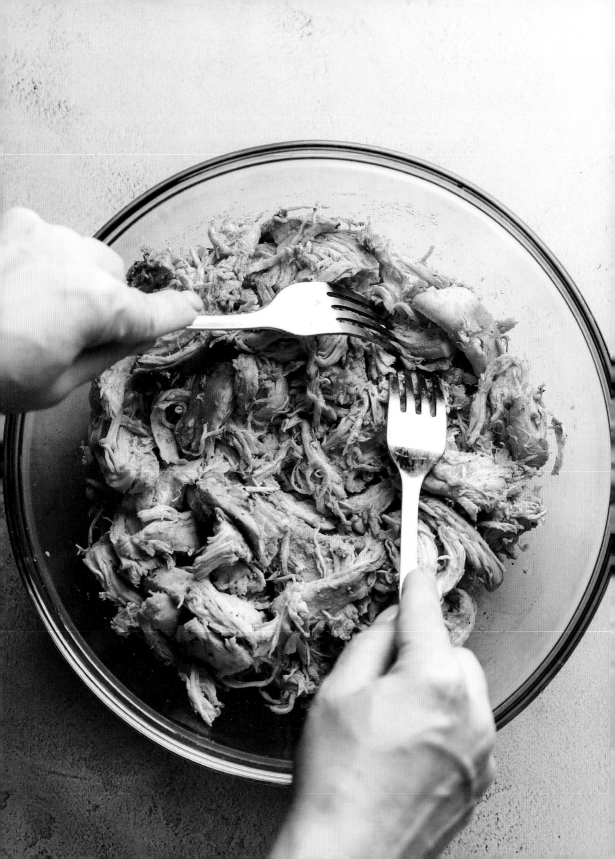

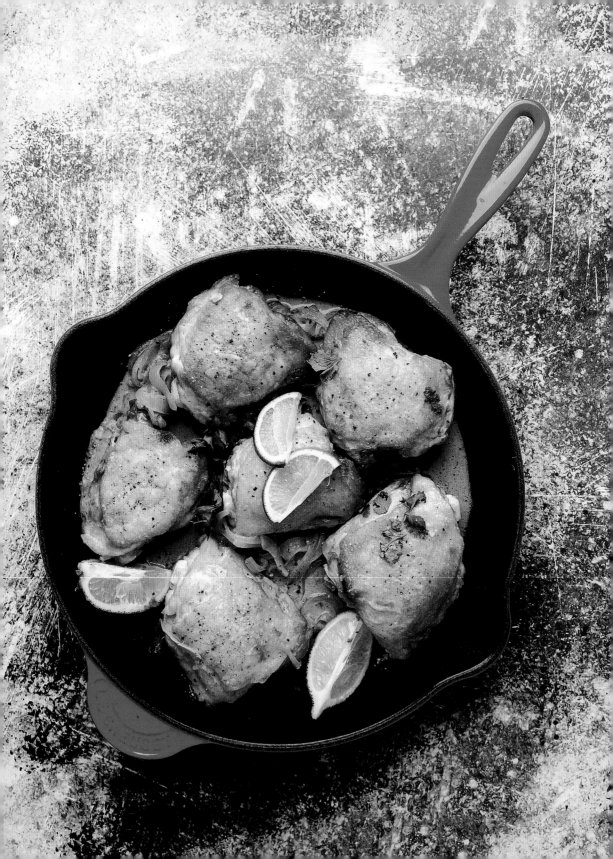

CURRY BRAISED CHICKEN THIGHS

Skin-on chicken thighs are budget-friendly and so juicy and full of flavor. Braised in a rich curry sauce, this chicken is excellent paired with the Turmeric Cauliflower Rice with Coconut on page 227!

Prep Time: 10 minutes | Cook Time: 40 minutes | Total Time: 50 minutes

6 whole bone-in and skin-on chicken thighs

Salt to taste

½ onion, thinly sliced

3 garlic cloves, minced

2 tablespoons minced fresh ginger or ginger paste

2 tablespoons curry powder

1 (13.4-ounce) can full-fat coconut milk

Fresh cilantro, for garnish

1. Preheat the oven to 300°F. Trim the excess skin from the chicken thighs and discard. Season the chicken thighs on both sides with salt.

2. Place a large oven-safe skillet with a tight-fitting lid over medium-high heat. Place the thighs in the hot skillet, skin-side down, to render the fat from the chicken skin. Let cook until the skin releases from the pan, about 5 minutes. Remove the chicken from the pan and set aside.

3. Remove all but about 1 tablespoon of fat from the pan. Add the onion and cook until soft, about 5 minutes. Stir in the garlic, ginger, and curry. Let cook for 1 minute longer until fragrant and then stir in the can of coconut milk. Scrape any brown bits from the bottom of the pan. Season with salt to taste.

4. Add the chicken back to the pan and cover with a lid. Place the skillet in the oven to finish cooking the chicken, about 30 minutes. Top with fresh cilantro.

Makes 6 servings | Per serving: Calories: 374, Fat: 28g, Total CARBS: 5g, Fiber: 2g, Protein: 34g

JAMBALAYA WITH CHICKEN, SHRIMP, AND ANDOUILLE SAUSAGE

Jambalaya is a one-pot Cajun and Creole dish of rice, shrimp, chicken, and vegetables. There are many variations on the dish, and now, I'll add my keto-friendly version! This brings all the smoky, tomatoey goodness of the Creole dish but swaps in cauliflower rice to cut the carbs.

Prep Time: 10 minutes | Cook Time: 35 minutes | Total Time: 45 minutes

2 tablespoons avocado oil

1 pound andouille sausage, sliced into 1-inch pieces

1 small onion, diced

1 red bell pepper, diced

2 celery stalks, thinly sliced

1 pound boneless, skinless chicken thighs, diced into bite-sized pieces

1 (15-ounce) can fire-roasted tomatoes

2 cups chicken broth

½ teaspoon dried thyme

2 teaspoons dried oregano

1 tablespoon Cajun seasoning

½ teaspoon cayenne pepper

Salt to taste

1 pound (13–15 ct) shrimp, peeled and deveined

12 ounces frozen cauliflower rice

1. Heat the oil in a large Dutch oven over medium-high heat. Add the sausage and brown on both sides, about 2 minutes per side. Remove from the pan and set aside.

2. Reduce the heat to medium and toss the onion, bell pepper, and celery into the pot. Sauté for 5–7 minutes, until the vegetables are soft. Add the chicken, tomatoes, broth, thyme, oregano, Cajun seasoning, and cayenne. Cover with a lid and cook for 15 minutes, stirring occasionally, until the chicken is cooked through. Season with salt to taste.

3. Stir in the shrimp and cauliflower rice and cook for 5 minutes, until the shrimp is opaque and the rice is heated through. Top with the sausage.

Makes 6 servings | Per serving: Calories: 521, Fat: 35g, Total CARBS: 8g, Fiber: 3g, Protein: 44g

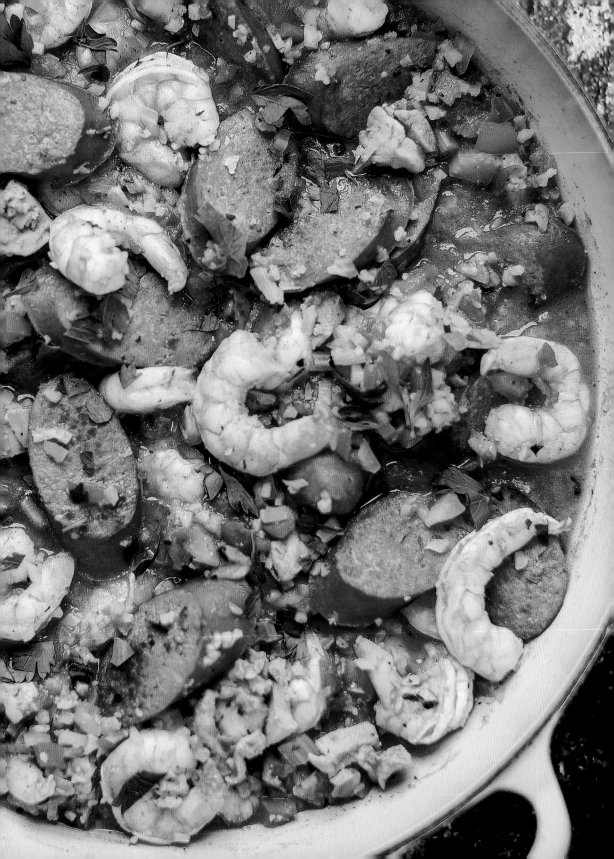

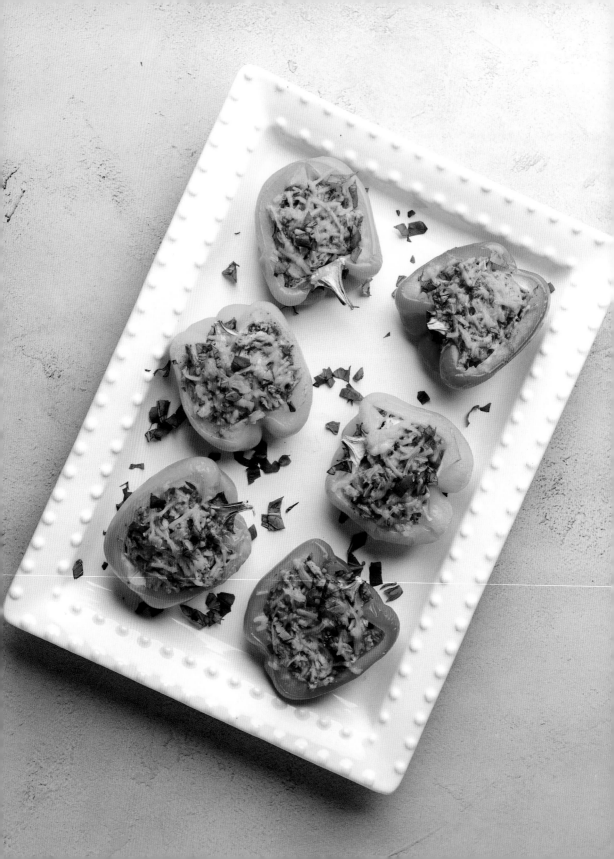

BBQ SHREDDED CHICKEN STUFFED PEPPERS

Stuffed peppers are such a classic, but filling them with BBQ chicken and cheese kicks them up a notch and gives them a fresh spin! Sugar-free BBQ sauce is an easy find in most grocery stores. My favorite brand is G Hughes. Use a store-bought rotisserie chicken for ease, or use my Shredded Chicken Breast recipe on page 142.

Prep Time: 10 minutes | Cook Time: 35 minutes | Total Time: 45 minutes

3 bell peppers, halved and seeds removed

3 cups cooked shredded chicken

2 cups shredded cheddar cheese, divided

¼ cup BBQ Dry Rub (page 254)

½ cup sugar-free BBQ sauce

1. Preheat the oven to 400°F and spray a 9 × 13–inch baking dish with cooking spray.

2. Place the halved bell peppers in a large microwave-safe bowl and microwave on high for 5 minutes to soften. Transfer to the prepared baking dish.

3. Combine the chicken, half of the shredded cheese, BBQ Dry Rub, and BBQ sauce in a large mixing bowl. Fill each bell pepper half with the shredded chicken mixture and top with the remaining cheese.

4. Bake for 30 minutes or until heated through and the cheese is bubbly.

Makes 6 servings | Per serving: Calories: 415, Fat: 25g, Total CARBS: 5g, Fiber: 1g, Protein: 42g

CHICKEN, BROCCOLI, AND CHEDDAR CASSEROLE

Pair chicken and a low-carb vegetable with a rich sauce and what's not to love? Maybe this easy and comforting casserole will get our kids to eat their vegetables!

Prep Time: 10 minutes | Cook Time: 40 minutes | Total Time: 50 minutes

2 tablespoons avocado oil

2½ pounds chicken breast, cut into 1-inch chunks

½ teaspoon kosher salt

¼ teaspoon pepper

1½ pounds fresh broccoli, cut into small florets

8 ounces cream cheese, softened

1 cup sour cream

2 chicken bouillon cubes, crumbled

2 cups shredded cheddar cheese

1. Preheat the oven to 350°F.

2. Heat the avocado oil in a large skillet over medium-high heat. Add the chicken to the pan and season with salt and pepper. Sauté until browned and cooked through, about 8 minutes.

3. Bring a large pot of salted water to a boil. Add the broccoli florets and cook, uncovered, until tender, 2 to 3 minutes. Drain.

4. Combine the cream cheese, sour cream, and bouillon in a large mixing bowl. Stir in the broccoli and cooked chicken. Pour into a 9 × 13–inch baking dish and top with the shredded cheese. Bake for 30 minutes, until heated through and bubbly.

Makes 8 Servings | Per serving: Calories: 492, Fat: 30g, Total CARBS: 6g, Fiber: 1g, Protein: 49g

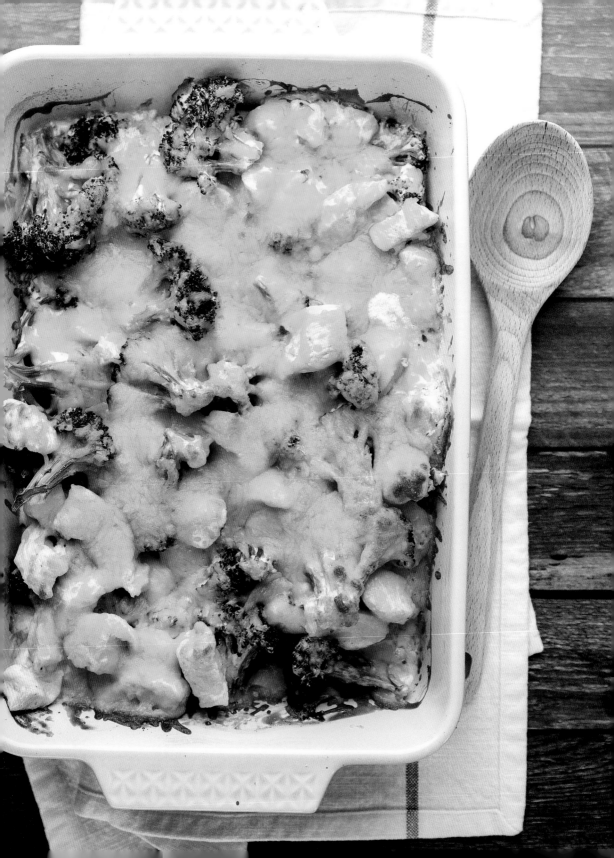

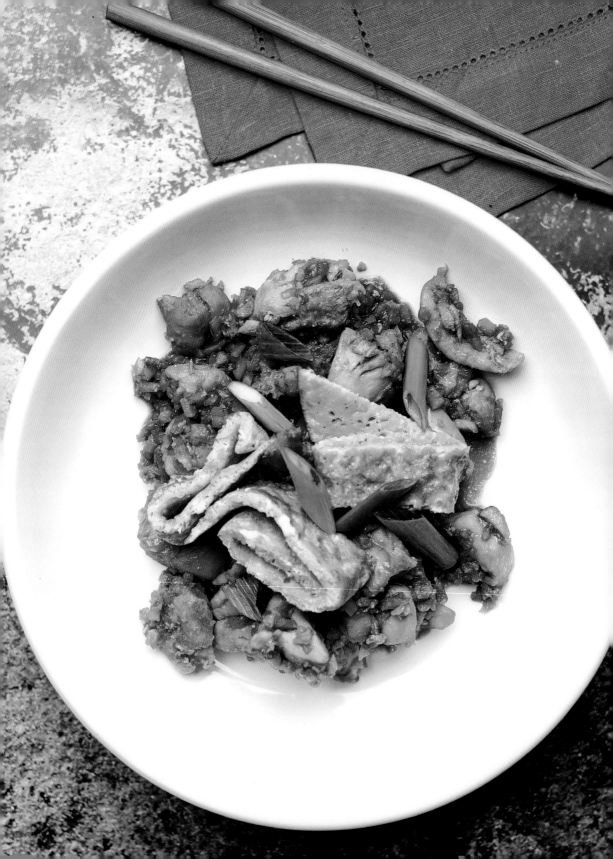

CHICKEN TERIYAKI FRIED RICE

Cauliflower rice is the perfect substitution to make an amazing keto-friendly chicken fried rice. I make my own delicious and easy teriyaki sauce right in the pan to pump up the flavor.

Prep Time: 10 minutes | Cook Time: 20 minutes | Total Time: 30 minutes

1 tablespoon avocado oil

2 pounds boneless, skinless chicken thighs, cut into bite-sized chunks

½ cup water

¼ cup soy sauce, tamari, or coconut aminos

3 tablespoons brown sugar sweetener

1 teaspoon grated fresh ginger or ginger paste

1 garlic clove, minced

¼ teaspoon xanthan gum

24 ounces cauliflower rice

4 large eggs

Sliced green onion for garnish

1. Heat the avocado oil in a large skillet over medium-high heat. Add the chicken to the pan and sauté for 5 minutes, until browned and cooked through. Stir in the water, soy sauce, brown sugar sweetener, ginger, garlic, and xanthan gum. Bring to a boil and cook until slightly thickened, about 3 minutes. Reduce the heat to medium-low and stir in the cauliflower rice.

2. While the rice is cooking, heat a small nonstick skillet over medium heat and spray with cooking spray. Two at a time, beat the eggs with a whisk or a fork in a small bowl, then cook in the skillet until cooked through, about 4 minutes. Remove from the pan to a cutting board and cut into strips.

3. Serve the fried rice topped with the sliced egg and green onion.

Makes 4 servings | Per serving: Calories: 423, Fat: 27g, Total CARBS: 6g, Fiber: 3g, Protein: 42g

CREAMY ITALIAN CHICKEN AND VEGETABLE SKILLET

This is my own creation, not an authentic Italian dish, but with the fragrant oregano and salty Parmesan, the flavors in this dish may just transport you to a quaint little restaurant in Italy. It is creamy, delicious, and packed with protein and veggies!

Prep Time: 10 minutes | Cook Time: 20 minutes | Total Time: 30 minutes

6 chicken breast cutlets

1 teaspoon oregano

Salt and pepper to taste

2 tablespoons avocado oil

3 tablespoons butter

3 cups baby spinach

2 cups cherry tomatoes, halved

1 crown broccoli, cut into small florets

3 garlic cloves, minced

1 cup heavy cream

2 ounces cream cheese

⅓ cup shredded Parmesan cheese

1. Season both sides of the chicken breast cutlets with the oregano, salt, and pepper.

2. Heat the avocado oil in a large skillet over medium-high heat. Sear both sides of the chicken breast cutlets, 2 minutes per side, until browned. Remove from the pan and set aside.

3. Reduce the heat to medium and melt the butter in the pan. Stir in the spinach, tomatoes, broccoli, and garlic. Season with salt and pepper. Let cook until the spinach is wilted, about 5 minutes. Stir in the heavy cream and cream cheese. Add the chicken back to the pan, cover with a lid, and cook for 10 minutes more or until broccoli is fork tender. Top with Parmesan cheese.

Makes 6 servings | Per serving: Calories: 442, Fat: 33g, Total CARBS: 5g, Fiber: 1g, Protein: 32g

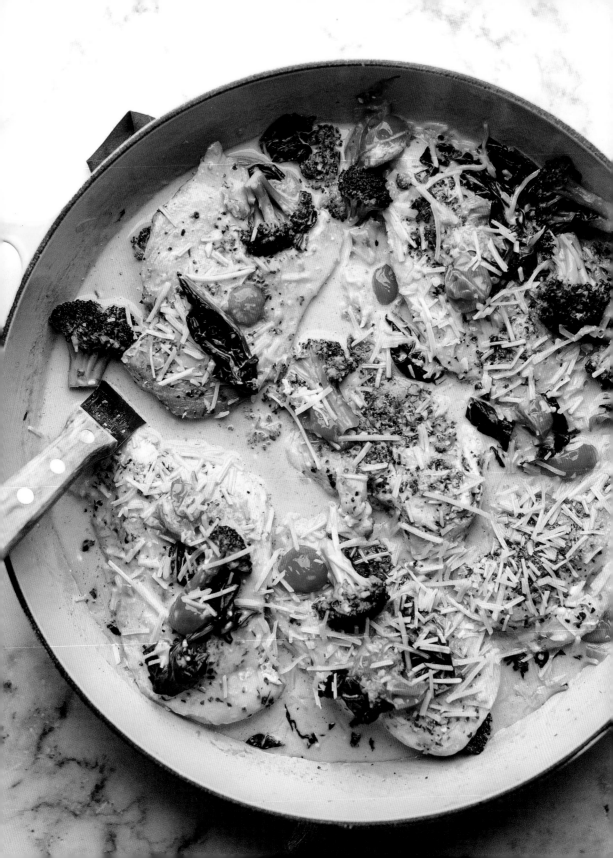

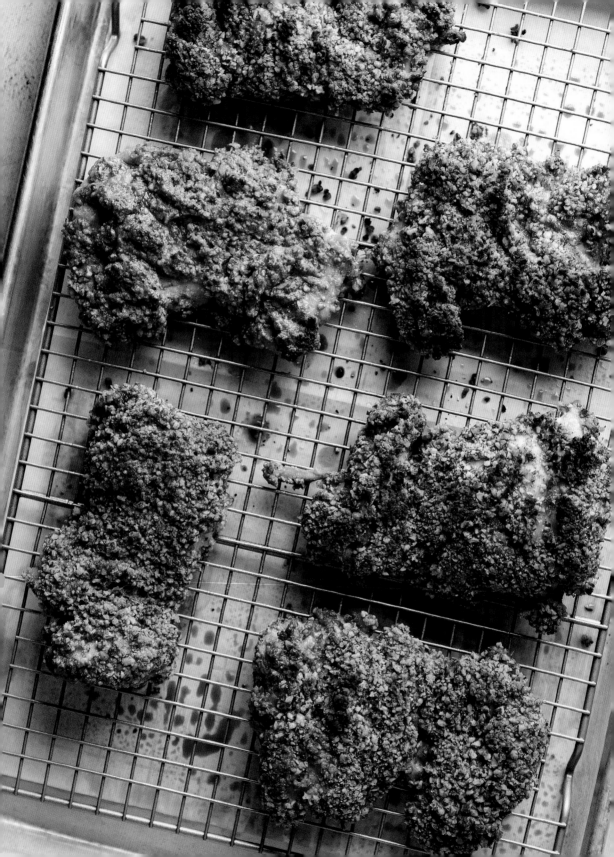

PECAN CRUSTED CHICKEN THIGHS

Crushed pecans make the perfect coating for chicken as they have such an amazing flavor, especially paired with Dijon mustard. You won't miss bland breadcrumbs!

Prep Time: 10 minutes | Cook Time: 20 minutes | Total Time: 30 minutes

1½ pounds boneless, skinless chicken thighs

¾ cup almond flour

3 large eggs

1 tablespoon Dijon mustard

2 cups finely chopped pecans

Salt and pepper to taste

1. Preheat the oven to 400°F. Spray a baking rack and rimmed baking sheet with cooking spray. Alternatively, you can line the baking sheet with foil for easy cleanup. Place the baking rack inside the baking sheet.

2. Create a breading station for the chicken: In a large shallow bowl, have ready your almond flour. In a second large shallow bowl, whisk together the eggs and Dijon mustard until well beaten. In a third large shallow bowl, spread the chopped pecans.

3. Season each chicken thigh with salt and pepper on both sides. Dredge a piece of chicken in the almond flour and coat completely, followed by the egg mixture to coat completely; finally, coat completely in the chopped pecans and place the chicken on the baking rack. Repeat this process with each piece of chicken.

4. Bake 20 minutes or until a thermometer inserted into the center of the chicken registers 165°F.

Makes 6 servings | Per serving: Calories: 403, Fat: 35g, Total CARBS: 3g, Fiber: 2g, Protein: 19g

CREAMY MUSHROOM GARLIC CHICKEN

Boneless, skinless chicken thighs are low in cost but high in flavor! In this dish, they pair up with a mushroom and garlic cream sauce that's just perfect for chilly fall and winter evenings. Serve with some mashed cauliflower, such as my Gruyère Mashed Cauliflower on page 228, for a warm and comforting meal.

Prep Time: 10 minutes | Cook Time: 25 minutes | Total Time: 35 minutes

1½ pounds boneless, skinless chicken thighs

Salt and pepper to taste

1 tablespoon avocado oil

1 pound baby bella mushrooms, sliced

½ teaspoon dried thyme

3 cloves minced garlic

¼ cup low-sodium chicken broth

¾ cup heavy cream

¼ cup grated Parmesan

1. Season the chicken thighs on both sides with salt and pepper.

2. Heat the avocado oil in a heavy-bottomed skillet over medium-high heat. Sear the chicken thighs just until browned, 2–3 minutes per side. Remove from the skillet and set aside.

3. Reduce the heat to medium. In the same skillet, sauté the mushrooms and thyme for 5 minutes or until soft. Stir in the garlic and cook for 1 minute more until fragrant.

4. Stir in the chicken broth and heavy cream. Bring to a boil, then reduce to a simmer and add the chicken back to the pan. Simmer for 10 minutes, until the chicken is cooked through. Garnish with grated Parmesan.

Makes 6 servings | Per serving: Calories: 296, Fat: 24g, Total CARBS: 3g, Fiber: 1g, Protein: 20g

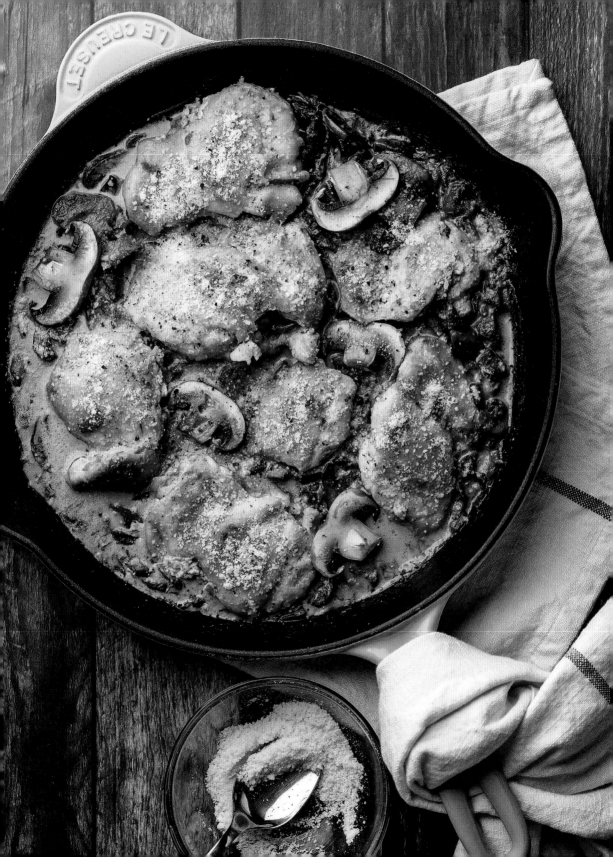

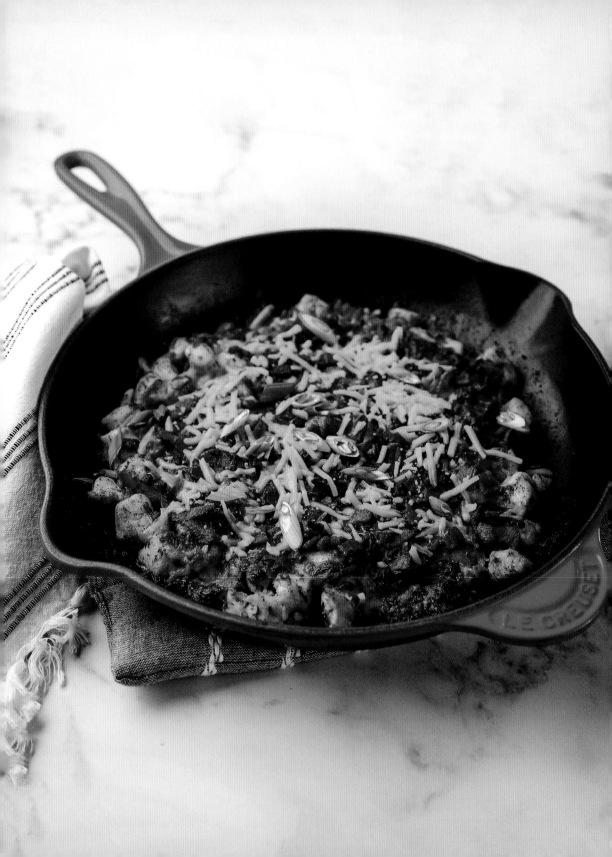

BACON RANCH CHICKEN SKILLET

What is not to love about bacon, ranch, and chicken? Cooking up the chicken in the rendered bacon fat gives it an extra savory note that just can't be beat. This is definitely one of my family's favorites, and I hope it becomes one of yours as well.

Prep Time: 5 minutes | Cook Time: 10 minutes | Total Time: 15 minutes

1 pound bacon, chopped

1½ pounds chicken breast, cut into bite-sized chunks

1 tablespoon dried parsley

1 teaspoon dried dill

1 teaspoon dried chives

1 teaspoon garlic powder

1 teaspoon onion powder

½ teaspoon kosher salt

¼ teaspoon pepper

1½ cups shredded cheddar cheese

1. In a heavy-bottomed skillet over medium-high heat, sauté the bacon for 10–15 minutes, or until crisp. Remove with a slotted spoon to a plate lined with paper towels and set aside to drain. Remove all but 2 tablespoons of the bacon fat from the pan.

2. Add the chicken and all seasonings to the pan and sauté until the chicken is browned and cooked through, about 8 minutes.

3. While the chicken cooks, preheat the oven to a high broil. When the chicken is cooked through, remove the skillet from the heat and top with the shredded cheddar cheese and the cooked bacon.

4. Place the skillet under the broiler on the middle rack until the cheese is melted and bubbly.

Makes 6 servings | Per serving: Calories: 398, Fat: 24g, Total CARBS: 2g, Fiber: 0g, Protein: 51g

FRENCH ONION CHICKEN ZOODLE SKILLET

Spiralized zucchini, or zoodles, make an excellent pasta replacement when you're craving noodles. While they do not taste exactly like traditional spaghetti, the texture and shape are reminiscent of pasta, and they give you a nice boost of veggies, too. In this dish, the French onion flavor really shines!

Prep Time: 10 minutes | Cook Time: 35 minutes | Total Time: 45 minutes

3 pounds zucchini, spiralized

½ teaspoon kosher salt

2 tablespoons avocado oil

1½ pounds boneless, skinless chicken thighs, cut into 1-inch chunks

Salt and pepper to taste

1 large onion, thinly sliced

½ teaspoon dried thyme

6 ounces provolone cheese, chopped

6 ounces provolone cheese, sliced

Makes 6 servings | Per serving: Calories: 429, Fat: 30g, Total CARBS: 11g, Fiber: 3g, Protein: 34g

1. Set a colander inside a larger bowl and fill with the zucchini noodles. Season the noodles with ½ teaspoon salt and let drain while you assemble the rest of the recipe.

2. Preheat the oven to high broil. Heat the oil in a large skillet over medium-high heat. Add the chicken to the pan and season with salt and pepper. Sauté the chicken for 8 minutes, until browned and cooked through. Remove from the pan and set aside.

3. Reduce the heat to medium. In the same pan, season the onions with thyme, salt, and pepper. Cook, stirring occasionally, until the onions are very soft and browned, about 20 minutes. If the onions are charring, reduce the heat.

4. Add the chicken, chopped cheese, and zucchini noodles to the pan with the onions and toss until well combined. Top with the sliced provolone cheese. Place under the broiler for 5 minutes or until the cheese is melted and slightly browned.

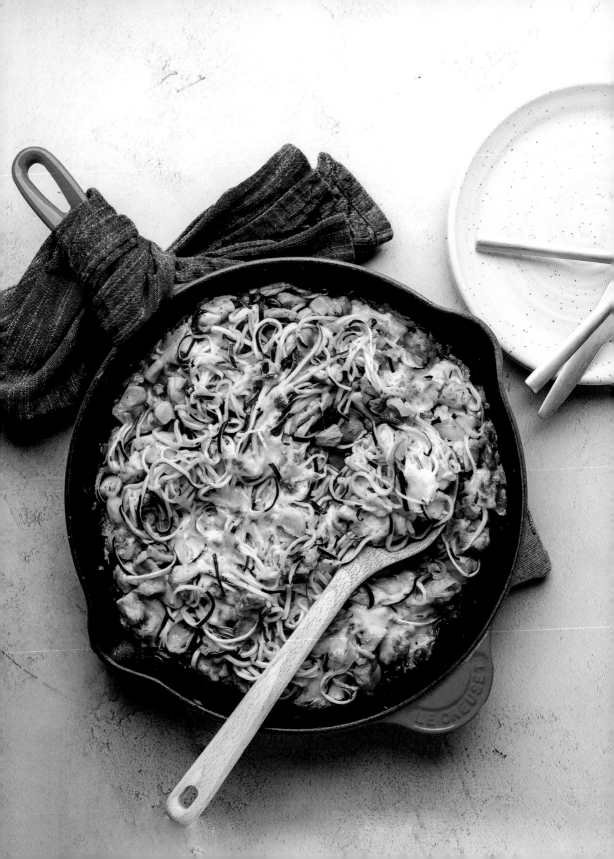

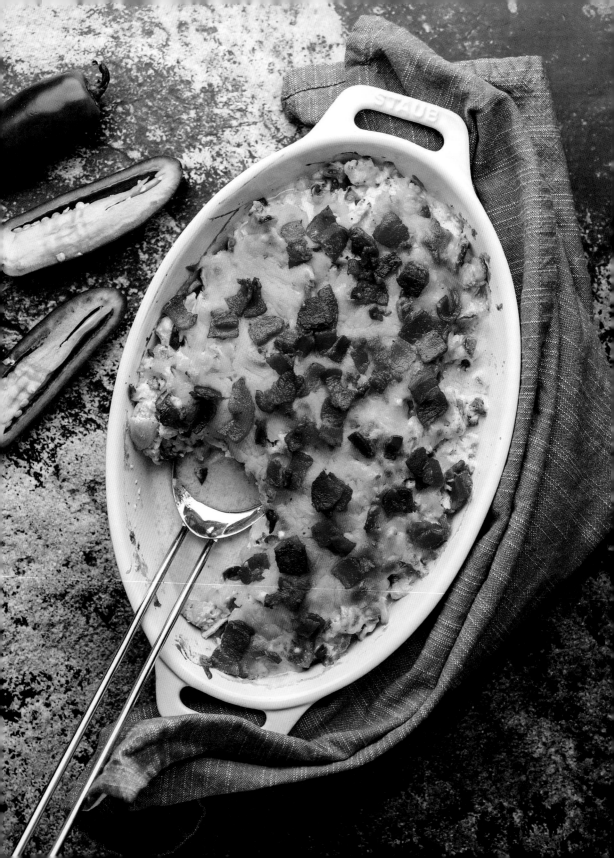

JALAPEÑO POPPER CHICKEN CASSEROLE

The flavor of the jalapeños in this casserole cannot be beat. If you like less heat, remove the seeds and you remove the spice. Problem solved! Using a rotisserie chicken is a great shortcut to get the shredded chicken for this recipe, or you can cook your own.

Prep Time: 10 minutes | Cook Time: 30 minutes | Total Time: 40 minutes

8 ounces cream cheese

½ cup heavy cream

¼ cup chicken broth

1 teaspoon garlic powder

1 teaspoon kosher salt

½ teaspoon pepper

5 ounces jalapeños, seeds removed and diced

2 pounds cooked shredded chicken

8 slices bacon, cooked and crumbled

1 cup shredded cheddar cheese

1. Preheat the oven to 400°F and spray a medium-sized casserole dish with cooking spray.

2. In a large mixing bowl, combine the cream cheese, heavy cream, chicken broth, garlic powder, salt, and pepper until well mixed. Stir in the jalapeños, chicken, and half of the bacon.

3. Pour into the casserole dish and top with the cheese and remaining bacon. Bake for 30 minutes or until the cheese is melted and bubbly.

Makes 6 servings | Per serving: Calories: 564, Fat: 38g, Total CARBS: 7g, Fiber: 1g, Protein: 49g

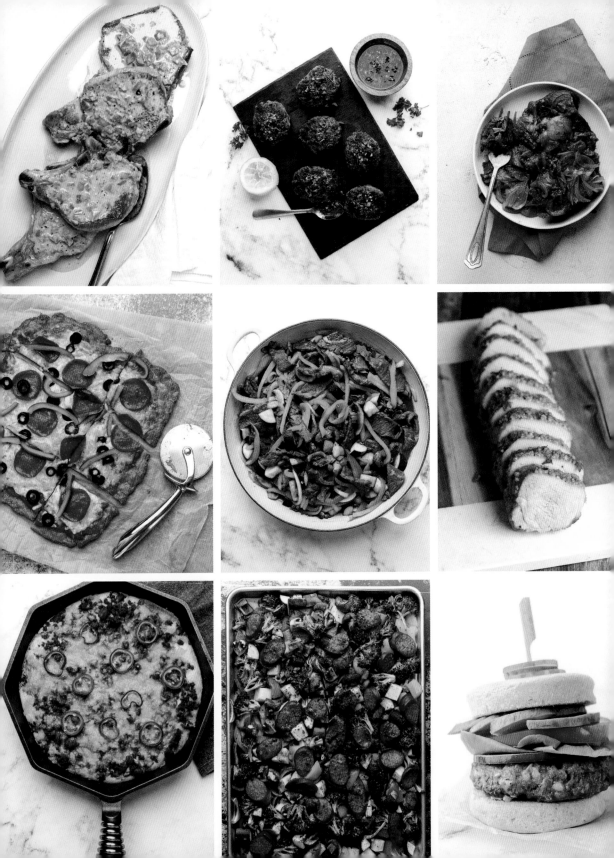

BEEF AND PORK

TACO "CORNBREAD"

I love quick family-friendly meals that use minimal cookware to prepare, and this Taco "Cornbread," made with just one skillet and one bowl, is a perfect example. Less mess means more time to spend with family! If you're not too fond of jalapeños, you can simply leave them off and dinner will be just as delicious.

Prep Time: 10 minutes | Cook Time: 30 minutes | Total Time: 40 minutes

1 pound ground beef

1½ teaspoons kosher salt

1½ teaspoons cumin

½ teaspoon garlic powder

½ teaspoon chili powder

½ teaspoon smoked paprika

2 cups almond flour

½ teaspoon baking powder

4 large eggs, beaten

1 cup half-and-half

1 cup shredded cheese

1 jalapeño, sliced (optional)

1. Preheat the oven to 350°F.

2. Place the ground beef in a large oven-safe skillet over medium-high heat and season with salt, cumin, garlic powder, chili powder, and paprika. Cook and crumble until browned, about 8 minutes.

3. In a large mixing bowl combine the almond flour and baking powder, followed by the eggs and half-and-half. Stir until well combined.

4. Pour over the ground beef and top with the shredded cheese. Top with the sliced jalapeños if you're using them. Bake for 30 minutes or until the cheese is melted and starting to brown.

Makes 6 servings | Per serving: Calories: 518, Fat: 40g, Total CARBS: 10g, Fiber: 4g, Protein: 32g

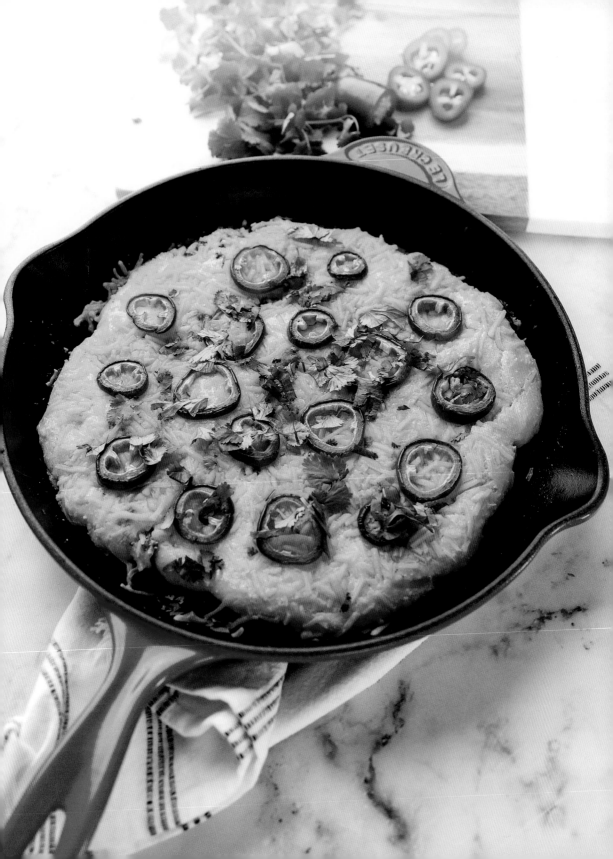

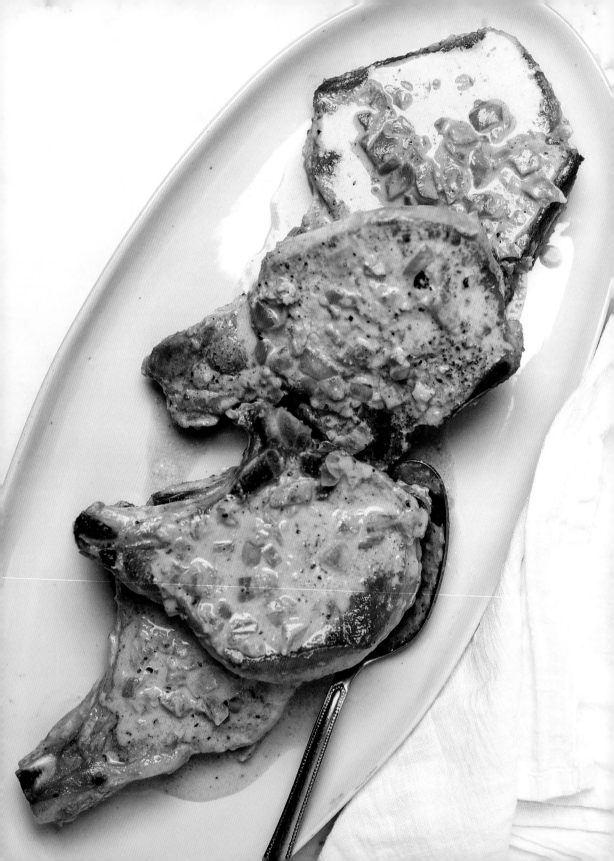

SMOTHERED PORK CHOPS

Smothered pork chops are a classic dish with many variations. In this version, tender chops are smothered in a simple onion cream sauce that is especially delicious served alongside green beans or steamed broccoli.

Prep Time: 10 minutes | Cook Time: 20 minutes | Total Time: 30 minutes

4 (8-ounce) bone-in pork chops

Salt and pepper to taste

½ teaspoon onion powder

½ teaspoon garlic powder

2 tablespoons avocado oil

½ cup diced onion

2 garlic cloves, minced

¾ cup heavy cream

½ cup chicken broth

1. Season both sides of the pork chops with salt, pepper, onion powder, and garlic powder.

2. Heat the oil in a large skillet over medium-high heat. Sear the pork chops for a few minutes on each side, until browned. Remove from the skillet and set aside.

3. Reduce the heat to medium and add the onion and garlic to the skillet. Cook until the onion is translucent, about 5 minutes.

4. Stir in the heavy cream and chicken broth. Add the pork chops back to the skillet and let simmer until the sauce slightly thickens and the pork chops are cooked through, about 10 minutes.

Makes 4 servings | Per serving: Calories: 546, Fat: 43g, Total CARBS: 3g, Fiber: 0g, Protein: 36g

BACON CHEESEBURGER MEATLOAF

If you need a hit with your family for dinner, this recipe might be a home run. My kids love anything with bacon, cheddar, and BBQ. Sugar-free BBQ sauce is now easy to find in most major grocery stores. My favorite brand is G Hughes.

Prep Time: 10 minutes | Cook Time: 50 minutes | Total Time: 1 hour

1 pound ground beef

½ pound bacon, cooked and crumbled

1 cup shredded cheddar cheese

1 large egg

1 teaspoon onion powder

1 teaspoon garlic powder

1 teaspoon mustard powder

1 teaspoon kosher salt

½ teaspoon pepper

⅓ cup sugar-free BBQ sauce

Sliced green onions, for garnish (optional)

1. Preheat the oven to 350°F and line a baking sheet with parchment paper or aluminum foil.

2. In a large mixing bowl, combine the ground beef, bacon, cheese, egg, onion powder, garlic powder, mustard powder, salt, and pepper. Mix well with your hands.

3. Turn the meat mixture out onto the prepared baking sheet and, with clean hands, form it into a 9 × 5–inch loaf shape.

4. Bake the meatloaf for 40 minutes, then remove from the oven and top with the BBQ sauce. Return to the oven for an additional 10 minutes. Slice and serve topped with green onions if you wish.

Makes 6 servings | Per serving: Calories: 405, Fat: 28g, Total CARBS: 2g, Fiber: 0g, Protein: 35g

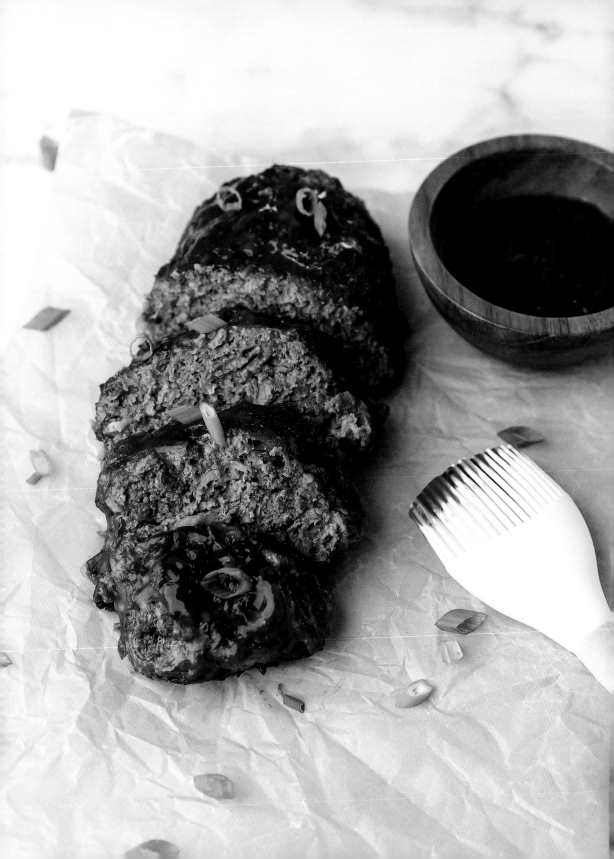

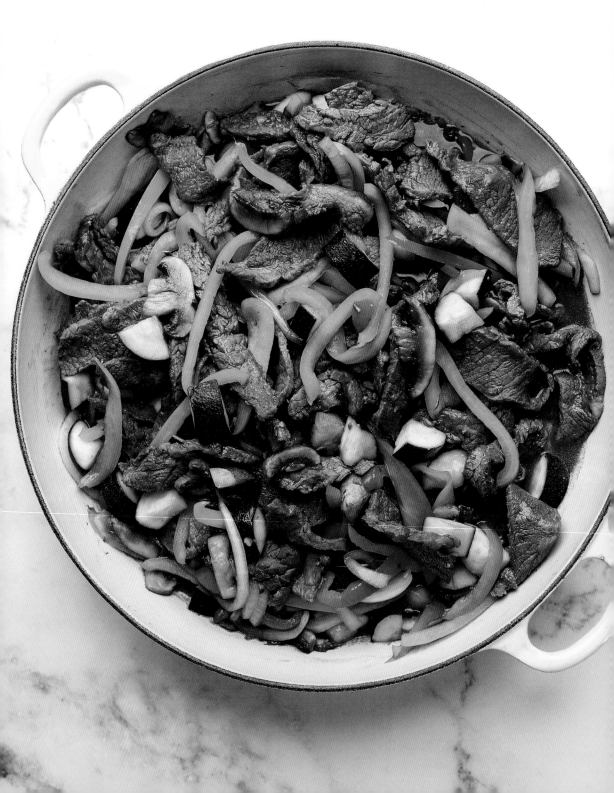

TERIYAKI BEEF AND VEGETABLE STIR-FRY

This veggie-forward dish brings a rainbow to your table! It is perfect as a quick weeknight dinner or split into individual servings for meal prep.

Prep Time: 10 minutes | Cook Time: 15 minutes | Total Time: 25 minutes

¼ cup soy sauce, tamari, or coconut aminos

3 tablespoons brown sugar sweetener

1 garlic clove, minced

1 teaspoon grated ginger

½ cup water

¼ teaspoon xanthan gum

2 tablespoons avocado oil

1½ pound flank steak or flatiron steak, cut thin against the grain

2 medium-sized zucchini, cut into chunks

1 red bell pepper, sliced

1 yellow bell pepper, sliced

1 green bell pepper, sliced

½ white onion, sliced thin

8 ounces baby bella mushrooms, sliced

1. Make the teriyaki sauce: In a medium mixing bowl whisk together the soy sauce, brown sugar sweetener, garlic, ginger, water, and xanthan gum. Set aside.

2. Heat the avocado oil in a large skillet over medium-high heat. Add the sliced steak to the skillet in a single layer and sear on both sides until browned, 2–3 minutes per side. Remove from the skillet and set aside.

3. Add all the vegetables to the skillet and cook, stirring frequently, until soft, about 5 minutes. Stir in the teriyaki sauce and bring the skillet to a simmer. Finally, add the steak back to the pan and toss just to evenly coat with the sauce. Serve immediately or divide the stir-fry among 4 airtight containers with tight-fitting lids and store in the fridge for up to 4 days. To reheat, microwave on high for 1½ minutes or until heated through.

Makes 4 servings | Per serving: Calories: 408, Fat: 21g, Total CARBS: 14g, Fiber: 4g, Protein: 43g

CARNIVORE PIZZA CRUST

Pork rinds make an amazing flour substitute in this keto pizza crust. Top this crust with your favorite toppings and pizza night lives on in your low-carb life!

Prep Time: 10 minutes | Cook Time: 20 minutes | Total Time: 30 minutes

1¾ cup shredded mozzarella cheese

1½ ounces crushed pork rinds

1 large egg

½ teaspoon Italian seasoning

Pinch of kosher salt

Your favorite pizza toppings

1. Preheat the oven to 400°F. Have ready a 12-inch square piece of parchment paper.

2. Combine the mozzarella cheese and crushed pork rinds in a large microwave safe bowl. Microwave on high for 1 minute or until the cheese is melted. Let the mixture cool for a few minutes.

3. When the mixture has cooled enough, stir in the egg and seasonings. Knead the dough with your hands until the egg is completely incorporated.

4. Turn the dough out onto the parchment paper and press into a round or rectangular crust ¼ inch thick. Place the parchment and pizza crust in the oven directly on the center rack and bake for 10 minutes. Pop any bubbles that form in the crust while baking.

5. Remove the parbaked crust from the oven and add your favorite pizza toppings. Bake for 8 minutes more or until the toppings are cooked to your liking.

Makes 4 servings | Per serving, crust only: Calories: 218, Fat: 16g, Total CARBS: 2g, Fiber: 0g, Protein: 21g

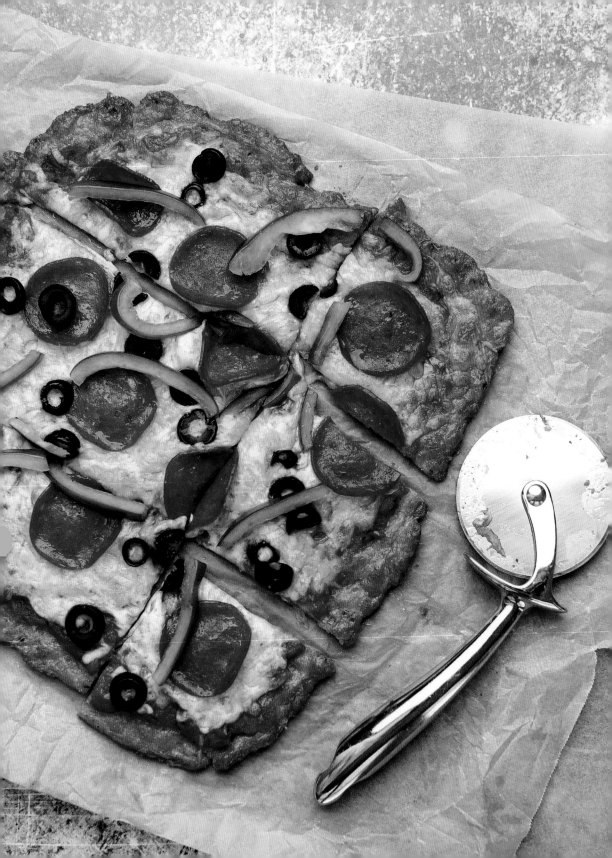

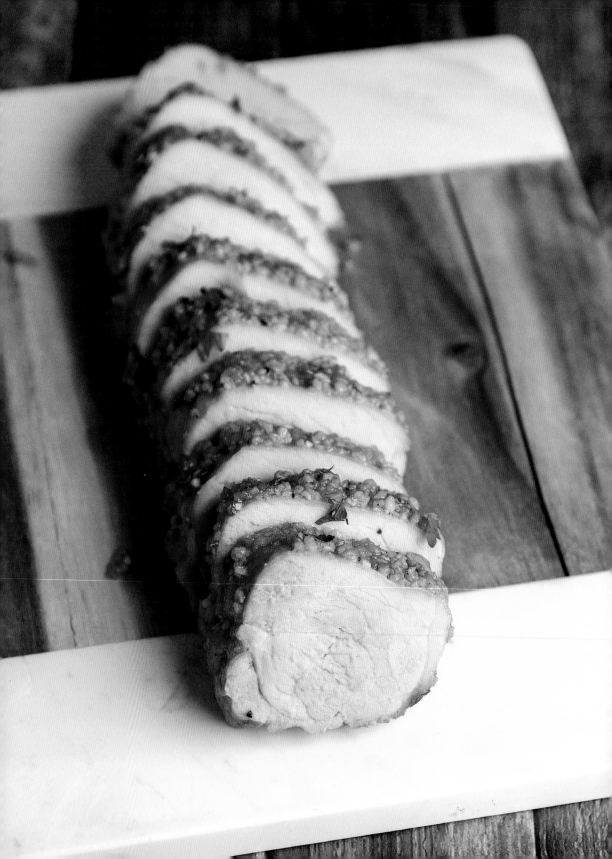

BROWN SUGAR GARLIC PORK TENDERLOIN

Trust me on this combo of brown sugar and garlic because it is amazing! The juicy pork pairs perfectly with the sweet and savory rub. I love to pair this dish with a simple vegetable sautéed in butter such as zucchini or green beans.

Prep Time: 5 minutes | Cook Time: 20 minutes | Total Time: 25 minutes

1½ pounds pork tenderloin

1 tablespoon avocado oil

¼ cup minced garlic

¼ cup brown sugar sweetener

1½ teaspoons kosher salt

½ teaspoon black pepper

Chopped fresh parsley, for garnish (optional)

1. Preheat the oven to 400°F and line a baking sheet with aluminum foil. Place the pork tenderloin on the baking sheet.

2. In a medium-sized mixing bowl combine the avocado oil, garlic, sweetener, salt, and pepper. Using a spoon, spread the garlic mixture on top of the pork tenderloin, coating evenly.

3. Bake for 20 minutes or until a meat thermometer inserted into the center reads 145°F. Remove to a cutting board and spoon the juices from the baking sheet over the tenderloin. Allow it to rest for 5–10 minutes before slicing into 1-inch pieces (resting helps keep the tenderloin juicy). Serve garnished with fresh chopped herbs if you like.

Makes 4 servings | Per serving: Calories: 295, Fat: 10g, Total CARBS: 3g, Fiber: 0g, Protein: 45g

BEEF TACO CUPS

Who needs tortillas to make taco night fun? Crispy cheddar cups are the new taco shells in my house! They are super easy to make and hold lots of delicious filling.

Prep Time: 10 minutes | Cook Time: 20 minutes | Total Time: 30 minutes

2 cups shredded cheddar cheese

1 pound ground beef

½ teaspoon onion powder

1½ teaspoon kosher salt

1½ teaspoon cumin

½ teaspoon chili powder

½ teaspoon smoked paprika

Your favorite taco toppings

1. Preheat the oven to 350°F and line a sheet tray with parchment paper.

2. Place 8 (¼-cup) piles of cheese evenly spaced on the sheet tray. Bake for 10 minutes or until the cheese is melted into rounds and just starting to brown around the edges. Remove from the oven and cool for 5 minutes, until the cheese is still bendable but cool enough to handle.

3. Peel the melted cheese off of the parchment paper and carefully place inside the cups of a muffin pan, making 8 taco cups. Let sit for 5 more minutes.

4. While the taco cups are cooling, make your beef taco meat. Heat a large skillet over medium-high heat. Cook and crumble the ground beef until cooked through, about 8 minutes. Stir in all of the seasonings and let the beef cook for a few minutes longer to meld the flavors.

5. To serve, take a cheese cup and fill with the taco meat, followed by your favorite taco toppings.

Makes 4 servings; 2 taco cups per serving | Per serving: Calories: 429, Fat: 30g, Total CARBS: 2g, Fiber: 0g, Protein: 35g

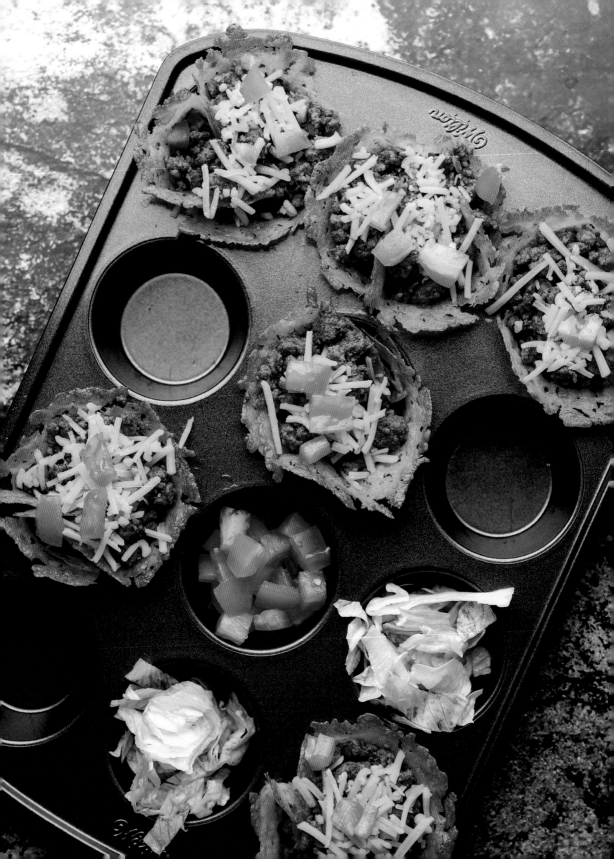

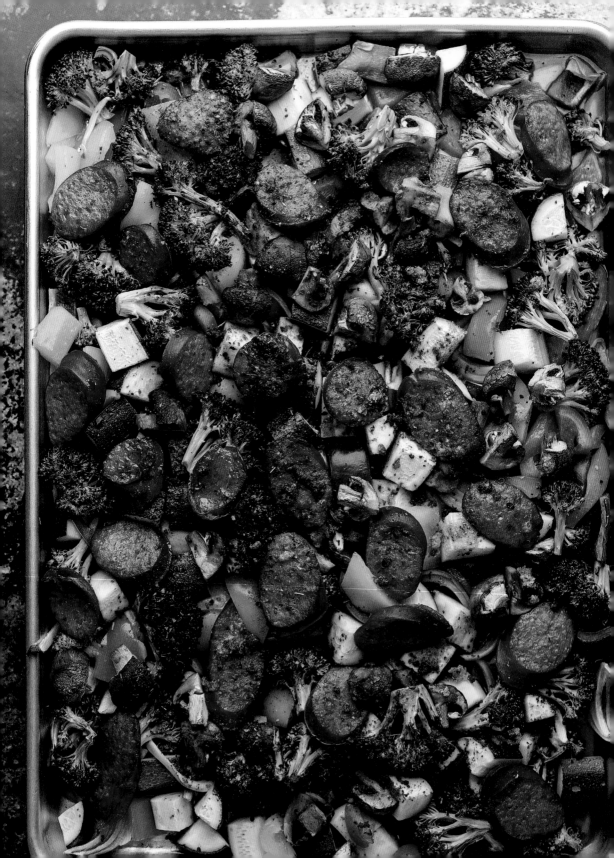

SHEET PAN SAUSAGE AND VEGGIES

I cannot get enough of this easy and delicious sheet pan meal loaded with veggies!
This recipe works perfectly for a quick dinner or as an easy lunch meal prep. Most
kielbasas are keto-friendly at only 2 grams of carbs per serving.

Prep Time: 10 minutes | Cook Time: 20 minutes | Total Time: 30 minutes

3 cups broccoli florets

8 ounces baby bella
mushrooms, quartered

1 red bell pepper, chopped

1 yellow bell pepper, chopped

1 green bell pepper, chopped

2 medium zucchini, cut into
1-inch chunks

½ red onion, sliced thin

½ cup avocado oil

2 teaspoons smoked paprika

2 teaspoons kosher salt

1 teaspoon dried oregano

1 teaspoon garlic powder

½ teaspoon black pepper

1 pound kielbasa sausage,
sliced into 1-inch slices

1. Preheat the oven to 425°F.

2. In a large mixing bowl combine all of the
vegetables with the avocado oil, paprika, salt,
oregano, garlic powder, and pepper. Stir until the
vegetables are well coated with the seasonings.

3. Pour onto a large rimmed baking sheet and top
with the sliced sausage. Bake for 20 minutes or
until the vegetables are fork tender. Serve right
away or divide the veggies and sausage among
6 airtight containers with tight-fitting lids.
Store in the fridge for up to 4 days. To reheat,
microwave on high for 1½ minutes or until
heated through.

Makes 6 servings | Per serving: Calories: 417, Fat: 34g, Total CARBS: 13g, Fiber: 4g, Protein: 16g

SWEET AND TANGY POT ROAST

The thought of this recipe simmering away on my stovetop on a cold Sunday afternoon has me excited for colder weather! A chuck roast is an excellent choice for pot roast because its higher fat content makes it super flavorful and tender after cooking low and slow.

Prep Time: 10 minutes | Cook Time: 2–3 hours | Total Time: 3 hours, 10 minutes

15 ounces canned tomato sauce

¼ cup brown sugar sweetener

2 tablespoons Worcestershire sauce

2 tablespoons apple cider vinegar

2 tablespoons avocado oil

2½ pounds chuck roast

Salt and pepper to taste

1 medium white onion, thinly sliced

Fresh-chopped parsley, for garnish (optional)

1. In a medium-sized mixing bowl, combine the tomato sauce, sweetener, Worcestershire sauce, and apple cider vinegar. Set aside.

2. Heat the avocado oil in a large-sized heavy-bottomed pot or Dutch oven over medium-high heat. Season all sides of your roast with salt and pepper. Sear the roast for 3 minutes on each side, until a brown crust forms. Top the seared roast with the onions and sauce mixture. Reduce the heat to low, cover with a lid, and let simmer for 2–3 hours or until the meat shreds easily with a fork.

3. Cut the roast into thick slices—it may fall apart a bit, and that's okay! Serve topped with the sauce and chopped fresh parsley if you wish.

Makes 6 servings | Per serving: Calories: 310, Fat: 13g, Total CARBS: 7g, Fiber: 1g, Protein: 41g

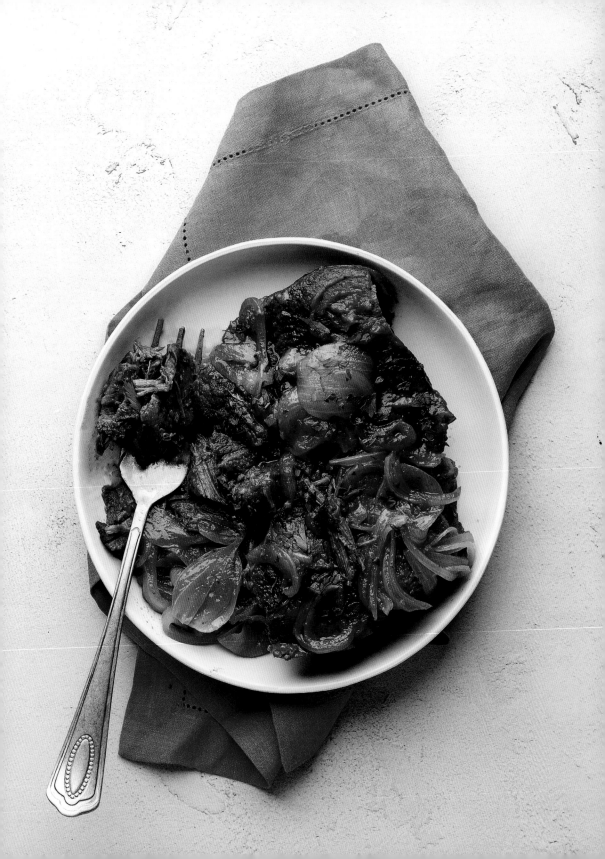

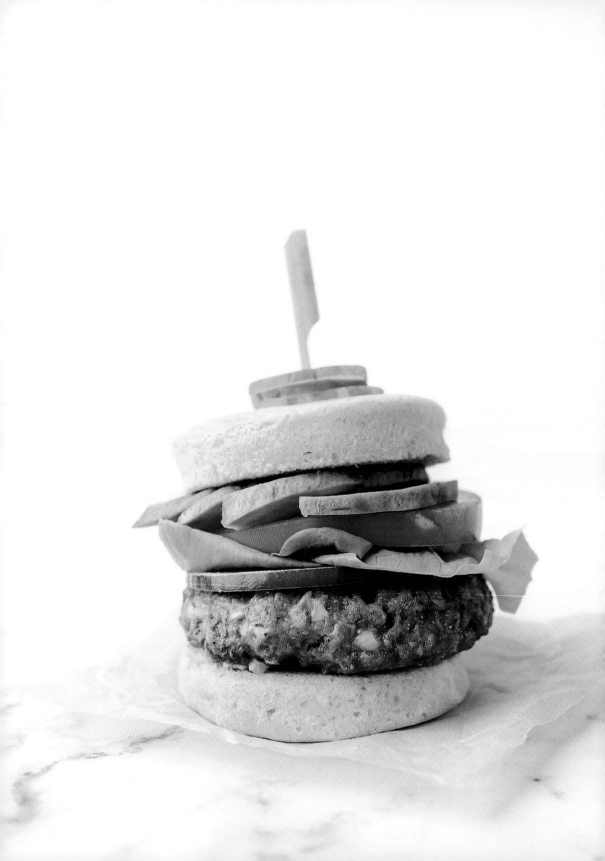

BEEF AND CHEDDAR BURGERS

Who doesn't love a good burger? The cheddar and onion right in the patties take the flavor to a new level. Serve them on keto bread (such as my Microwave Bread on page 257) or lettuce wraps with your favorite toppings!

Prep Time: 10 minutes | Cook Time: 10 minutes | Total Time: 20 minutes

1½ pounds ground beef

1 cup shredded cheddar cheese

1 small onion, finely minced

1 large egg, beaten

1 tablespoon Worcestershire sauce

½ teaspoon kosher salt

½ teaspoon black pepper

2 tablespoons avocado oil

1. Using your hands, combine all of the ingredients except the avocado oil in a large mixing bowl. Divide the mixture into 6 equal portions and shape into round patties.

2. Heat the avocado oil in a large skillet over medium-high heat. Cook the patties to your desired doneness, working in batches so as not to crowd the pan. Cook for 4 minutes on each side or until a meat thermometer inserted in the center registers 160°F. Serve immediately.

Makes 6 servings | Per serving (burgers only): Calories: 336, Fat: 24g, Total CARBS: 2g, Fiber: 0g, Protein: 28g

CHIMICHURRI KOFTA

Kofta is traditionally a Middle Eastern dish made with ground lamb or beef, shaped into logs or balls, grilled, and then served with pita or a sauce. Chimichurri sauce is a South American condiment that's made from oil and parsley and often used alongside barbecued meats. The pairing just works! Here, the chimichurri does double duty as the flavoring for the kofta and as a sauce for extra-easy prep.

Prep Time: 10 minutes | Cook Time: 15 minutes | Total Time: 25 minutes

½ cup + 2 tablespoons avocado oil, divided

Juice of 1 lemon

½ cup finely chopped parsley

4 garlic cloves, minced

1 teaspoon dried red pepper flakes

1 teaspoon kosher salt, divided

½ teaspoon dried oregano

1½ pounds ground beef

1. Make the chimichurri: In a small mixing bowl, whisk together ½ cup avocado oil, the lemon juice, parsley, garlic, red pepper flakes, ½ teaspoon salt, and oregano.

2. In a large mixing bowl combine the ground beef, remaining ½ teaspoon salt, and half of the chimichurri. Combine well with your hands. Divide into 6 equal portions and form each into a loaf shape.

3. Heat the remaining 2 tablespoons oil in a large skillet over medium-high heat. Sear the kofta for 4 minutes on each side. Serve with remaining chimichurri sauce.

Makes 6 servings | Per serving: Calories: 414, Fat: 35g, Total CARBS: 1g, Fiber: 0g, Protein: 23g

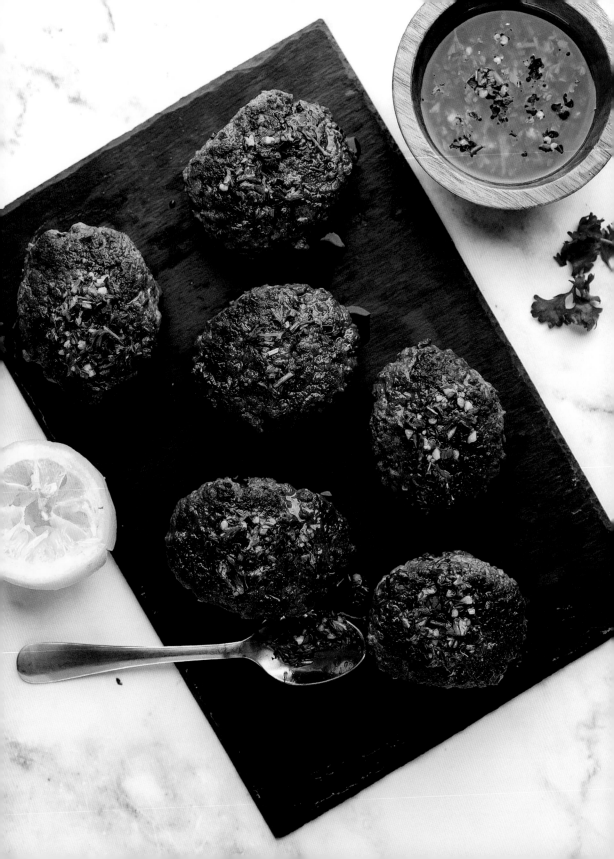

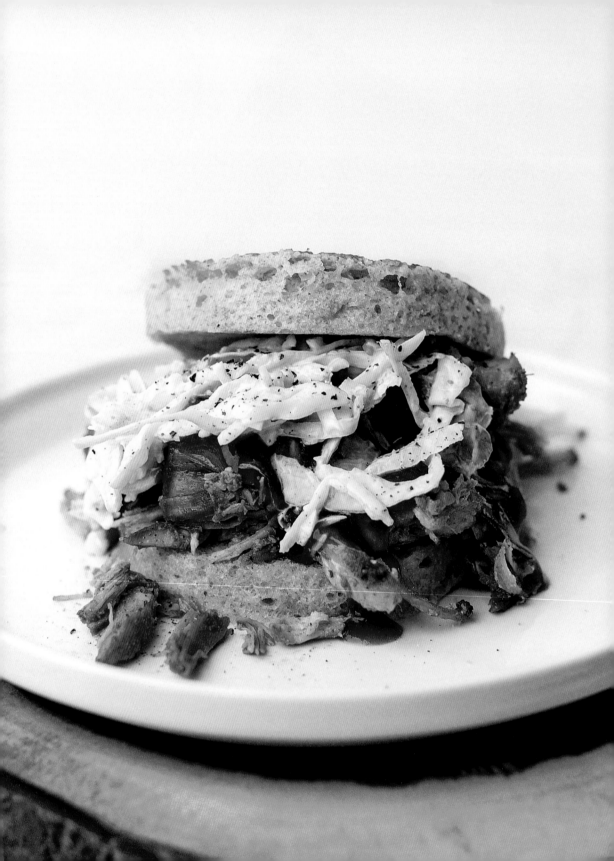

PULLED PORK SANDWICHES

There's just nothing like a pulled pork sandwich with tangy, sweet BBQ sauce and topped with a bright and acidic coleslaw. Use my BBQ Dry Rub, Microwave Bread, and Crunchy Coleslaw (pages 254, 257, and 231) to make all your BBQ dreams come true.

Prep Time: 10 minutes | Cook Time: 2 hours, 10 minutes | Total Time: 2 hours, 20 minutes

3 pounds boneless pork shoulder, pork butt, or picnic roast, cut into large chunks

¼ cup BBQ Dry Rub (page 254)

2 tablespoons avocado oil

1 cup water

BBQ Sandwiches

8 Microwave Breads (page 257) or lettuce leaves

1 batch Crunchy Coleslaw (page 231)

1 cup sugar-free BBQ sauce

1. In a large mixing bowl, use tongs to combine the pork chunks with the BBQ Dry Rub.

2. Heat the oil in a large-sized heavy-bottomed pot or Dutch oven over medium-high heat. Sear the pork chunks for 2 minutes on each side or until a brown crust forms. Add the water to the pot and use a wooden spoon to scrape any burnt bits from the bottom of the pan. Reduce the heat to a simmer, cover with a lid, and cook for 2 hours or until the pork shreds easily with a fork.

3. Have ready the Microwave Breads or lettuce wraps, Crunchy Coleslaw, and your favorite sugar-free BBQ sauce. Transfer the pulled pork to a serving bowl or platter to let everyone assemble their own sandwiches.

Makes 8 servings | Per serving, pork, slaw, and 2 tablespoons BBQ sauce only: Calories: 413, Fat: 21g, Total CARBS: 5g, Fiber: 1g, Protein: 47g

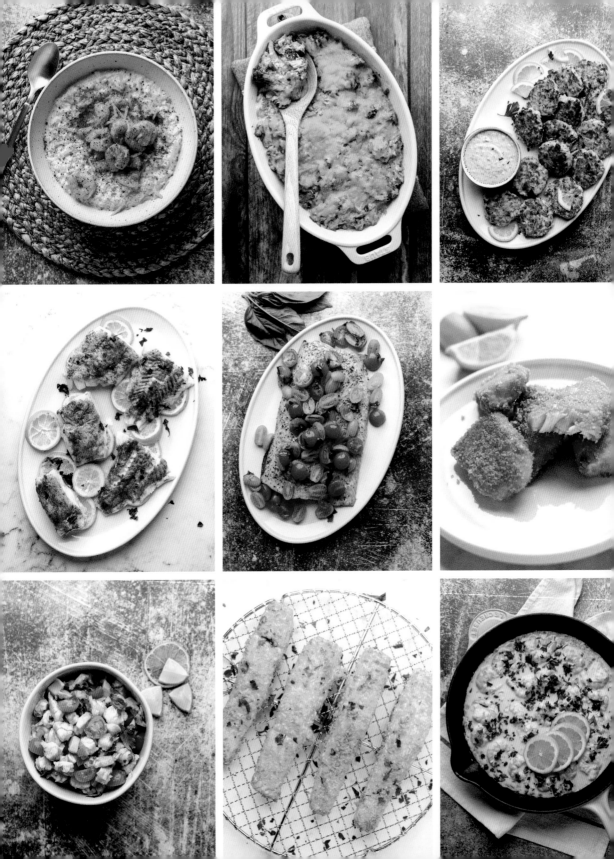

SEAFOOD

GARLIC BUTTER SHRIMP AND CAULI GRITS

As a southern girl, I had to create a keto-friendly version of this iconic southern dish. Can you believe frozen cauliflower rice pulsed in a food processor makes a spot-on substitute for grits? The richness from the butter and cheese and the hint of heat from the spices really take this to the next level. This dish is perfect for an indulgent brunch or dinner.

Prep Time: 10 minutes | Cook Time: 10 minutes | Total Time: 20 minutes

2 (12-ounce) bags frozen cauliflower rice, cooked according to package directions

7 tablespoons butter, divided

½ cup heavy cream

1 cup shredded cheddar cheese

4 garlic cloves, minced

1 pound jumbo shrimp, peeled and deveined

1½ teaspoons kosher salt

¼ teaspoon cayenne pepper

½ teaspoon garlic powder

½ teaspoon paprika, plus more for garnish

Black pepper to taste

1. Use a food processor to pulse the cooked cauliflower rice until it resembles coarse sand in consistency.

2. Heat the cauliflower, 3 tablespoons butter, and the heavy cream in a medium saucepan over medium heat until heated through. Stir in the cheese. Reduce the heat to low to keep warm.

3. Melt the remaining 4 tablespoons butter in a large skillet over medium heat. Stir in the garlic and cook until fragrant, about 1 minute. Add the shrimp to the pan and season with salt, cayenne, garlic powder, and paprika. Cook until the shrimp is opaque, stirring occasionally, about 4 minutes.

4. Serve the grits topped with the garlic butter shrimp. Garnish with a sprinkle of paprika and some pepper if you like.

Makes 4 servings | Per serving: Calories: 571, Fat: 44g, Total CARBS: 11g, Fiber: 4g, Protein: 39g

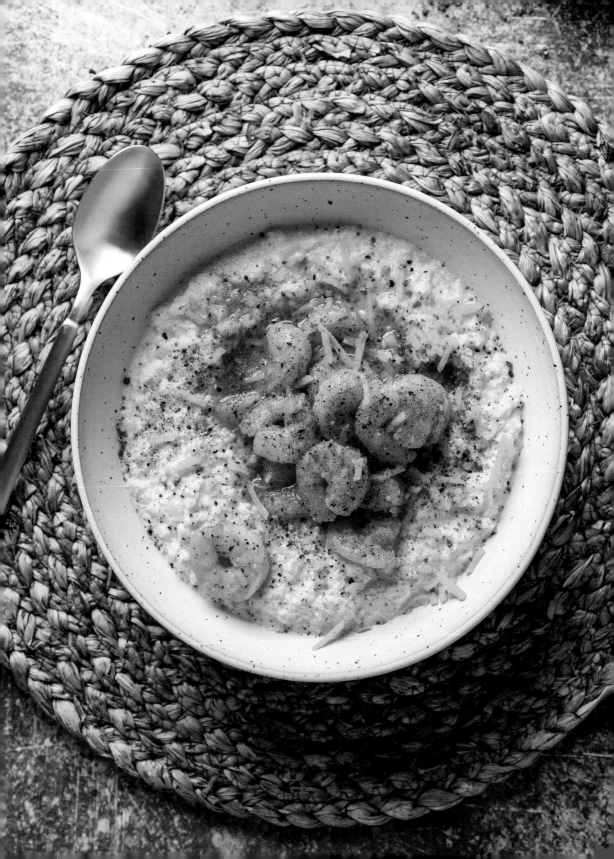

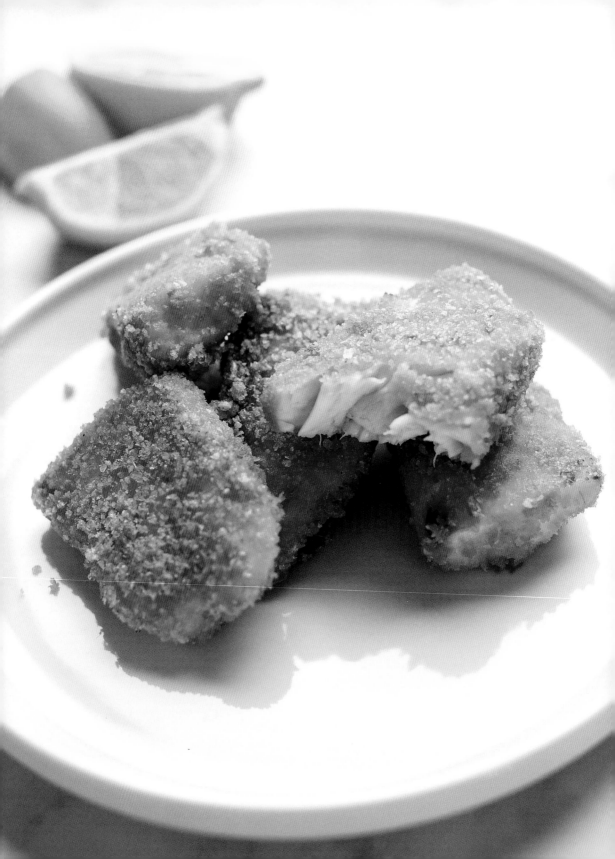

CRISPY BAKED FISH

Crushed pork rinds (fried pork skins) are a savory keto-friendly replacement for breadcrumbs. Actually, I like them better! You can pick up a bag of pork rinds in most grocery stores and pulse them in the food processor, or you can sometimes buy them already crushed! This recipe brings all the appeal of fried fish but without the carbs. Don't forget the lemon wedges to squeeze on top!

Prep Time: 10 minutes | Cook Time: 20 minutes | Total Time: 30 minutes

2 large eggs

2 tablespoons water

1½ ounces pork rinds, crushed

½ teaspoon garlic powder

½ teaspoon onion powder

½ teaspoon kosher salt

4 (4–6 ounce) white fish filets (such as tilapia or cod), cut into quarters

1. Preheat the oven to 425°F and line a baking sheet with parchment paper.

2. Create your breading station: Beat together the eggs and water in a shallow bowl. In a separate shallow bowl, combine the crushed pork rinds and seasonings.

3. Dip one piece of fish in the egg, followed by the pork rinds, coating the filet completely. Place on the baking sheet and repeat the process with the remaining pieces of fish.

4. Bake for 20 minutes until the exterior is golden and crispy, flipping halfway through.

Makes 4 servings | Per serving: Calories: 217, Fat: 11g, Total CARBS: 1g, Fiber: 0g, Protein: 31g

SHRIMP CAKES WITH CAJUN AIOLI

Everyone has heard of crab cakes, but have you tried shrimp cakes? Shrimp are a great budget-friendly alternative to the popular crab and just as delicious. The spicy and acidic aioli really gives a nice kick to the rich shrimp cakes. Mincing shrimp is a cinch—you can chop finely with a knife or pulse in a food processor.

Prep Time: 15 minutes | Cook Time: 20 minutes | Total Time: 35 minutes

1½ cups almond flour

¼ cup diced celery

½ red bell pepper, diced

1 teaspoon Creole seasoning

¼ teaspoon kosher salt

2 tablespoons chopped fresh parsley

1 pound raw peeled and deveined shrimp, minced

2 large eggs, beaten

2½ tablespoons mayonnaise

1½ teaspoons Dijon mustard

1 teaspoon Worcestershire sauce

2 tablespoons avocado oil

Cajun Aioli

1 cup mayonnaise

3 tablespoons dill pickle relish

2 teaspoons Dijon mustard

2 tablespoons minced white onion

2 tablespoons lemon juice

1 teaspoon Creole seasoning

½ teaspoon dried dill

Kosher salt and pepper to taste

1. In a large mixing bowl combine the almond flour, celery, bell pepper, Creole seasoning, salt, and parsley. Stir in the shrimp, eggs, mayonnaise, Dijon mustard, and Worcestershire. Mix well. Form the mixture into 12–14 cakes and set aside on a baking sheet.

2. Heat the avocado oil in a large skillet over medium-high heat. Fry the shrimp cakes in 2 batches for a few minutes on each side, or until golden brown and a meat thermometer inserted in the center reads 160°F.

3. In a small bowl, combine all of the ingredients for the aioli. Serve the shrimp cakes topped with aioli.

Makes 6 servings; 2 shrimp cakes and 3 tablespoons sauce per serving | Per serving: Calories: 575, Fat: 45g, Total CARBS: 8g, Fiber: 3g, Protein: 17g

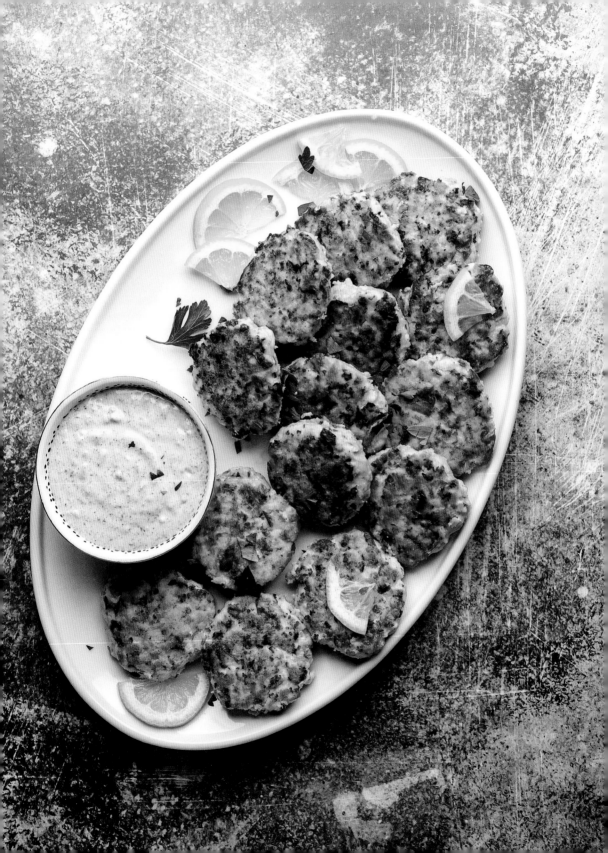

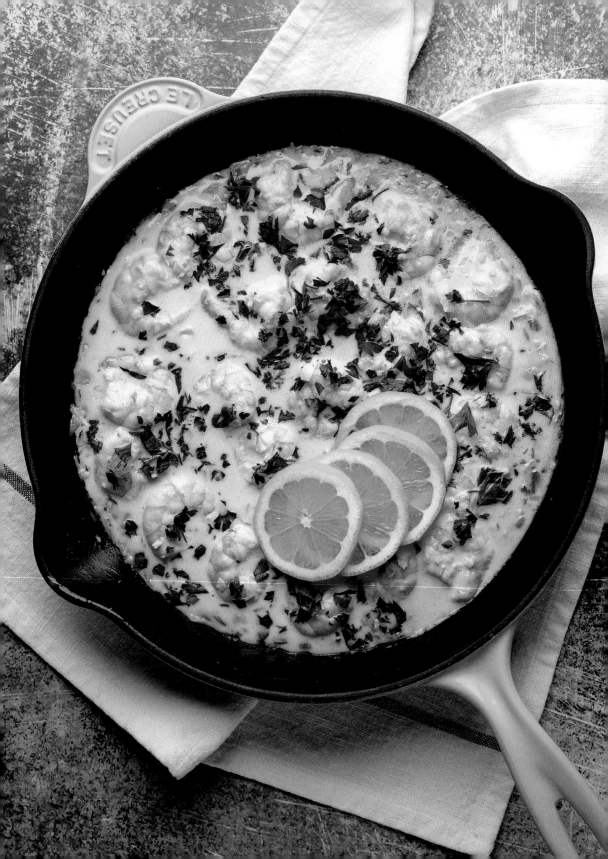

CREAMY SHRIMP SCAMPI

This quick shrimp dish makes a perfect weeknight dinner. Serve it with steamed spaghetti squash or zucchini noodles for a complete meal.

Prep Time: 10 minutes | Cook Time: 20 minutes | Total Time: 30 minutes

4 tablespoons butter, divided

½ medium onion, diced

6 garlic cloves, minced

½ cup chicken broth

Juice of one lemon

½ cup heavy cream

¼ cup grated Parmesan cheese

¼ teaspoon red pepper flakes

Salt to taste

1 pound large shrimp, peeled and deveined

¼ cup minced parsley

1. Melt 2 tablespoons of butter in a large skillet over medium heat. Stir in the onion and garlic and cook until translucent, about 5 minutes.

2. Stir in the chicken broth and lemon juice. Reduce the heat to medium-low and let simmer until reduced by half.

3. Stir in the heavy cream, Parmesan, red pepper flakes, and the remaining 2 tablespoons butter. Season with salt to taste. Add the shrimp, stirring to coat, and let cook for a few minutes, just until the shrimp is cooked through and opaque. Top with the minced parsley.

Makes 4 servings | Per serving: Calories: 383, Fat: 25g, Total CARBS: 7g, Fiber: 0g, Protein: 31g

TUNA AND BROCCOLI CASSEROLE

What better way to make this classic dish a bit healthier than to replace the pasta with broccoli? Frozen broccoli florets make for easier prep and a quicker cook time. If you want to use fresh, blanch the florets in boiling water for a couple of minutes before baking in the casserole.

Prep Time: 10 minutes | Cook Time: 30 minutes | Total Time: 40 minutes

12 ounces frozen broccoli florets, thawed

4 (5-ounce) cans tuna in water, drained

2 cups shredded cheddar cheese, divided

¾ cup mayonnaise

½ cup finely minced onion

2 tablespoons Dijon mustard

1 teaspoon kosher salt

½ teaspoon black pepper

½ teaspoon cayenne pepper

1. Preheat the oven to 350°F and spray a 9 × 13–inch casserole dish with cooking spray.

2. In a large mixing bowl, combine all the ingredients except for 1 cup of the cheddar cheese. Pour the mixture into the prepared baking dish and top with the remaining cheese.

3. Bake for 30 minutes or until the cheese is melted and starting to brown.

Makes 6 servings | Per serving: Calories: 448, Fat: 38g, Total CARBS: 8g, Fiber: 2g, Protein: 25g

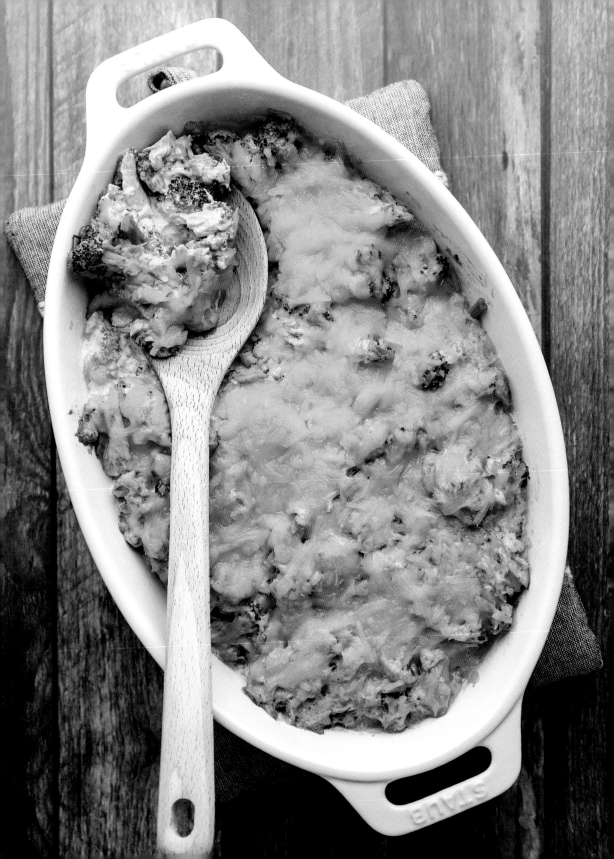

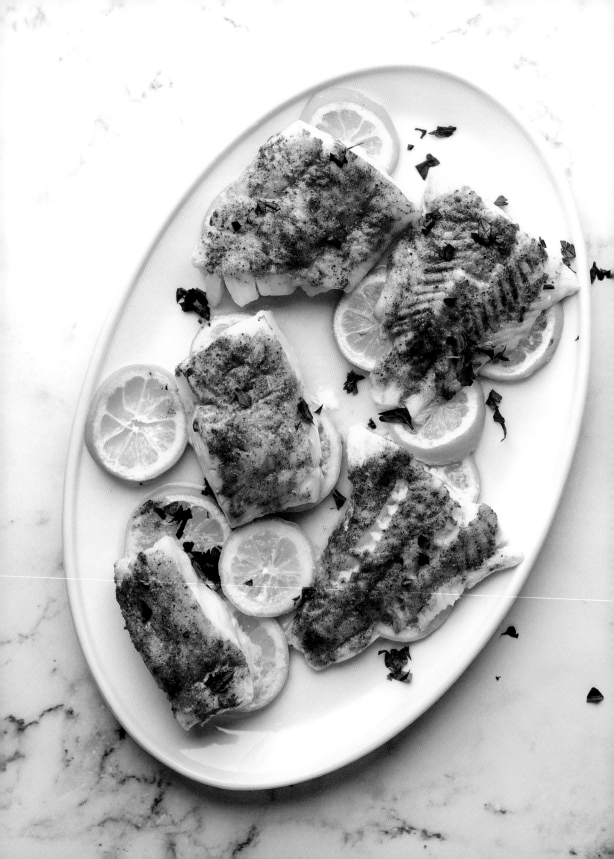

LEMON PEPPER COD

This classic flavor combination pairs perfectly with the mild cod fish. This is one of those recipes you could serve to company as it is very quick and looks stunning.

Prep Time: 5 minutes | Cook Time: 10 minutes | Total Time: 15 minutes

2 tablespoons lemon juice

½ teaspoon kosher salt

½ teaspoon pepper

½ teaspoon garlic powder

½ teaspoon paprika

2 lemons, sliced

6 (6-ounce) cod filets

Chopped fresh parsley, for garnish (optional)

1. In a small mixing bowl, whisk together the lemon juice, salt, pepper, garlic powder, and paprika. Set aside.

2. Preheat the oven to high broil and line a baking sheet with foil. Spray the foil with cooking spray.

3. Lay the sliced lemons on the baking sheet and place the cod filets on top. Use a basting brush to brush the seasoning over the cod filets. Place in the center of the oven and broil for 10 minutes or until the fish is slightly browned and flaky. Garnish with parsley if you like.

Makes 6 servings | Per serving: Calories: 135, Fat: 1g, Total CARBS: 6g, Fiber: 2g, Protein: 28g

BRUSCHETTA SALMON

A play on the classic Italian appetizer, this bruschetta salmon is easy enough for a weeknight meal but could also serve as a beautiful dish for a party. The brightness of the tomatoes really pairs well with the fatty salmon.

Prep Time: 10 minutes | Cook Time: 10 minutes | Total Time: 20 minutes

2 pounds salmon filets

2 tablespoons avocado oil

1 teaspoon Italian seasoning

1 teaspoon kosher salt

½ teaspoon pepper

Bruschetta Topping

10 ounces red cherry tomatoes, sliced in half lengthwise

10 ounces yellow cherry tomatoes, sliced in half lengthwise

6 basil leaves, roughly chopped

2 tablespoons avocado oil

2 tablespoons balsamic vinegar

Kosher salt and pepper to taste

1. Heat the oven to high broil and line a sheet tray with foil. Place the salmon on the foil, coat with the avocado oil, and season with the Italian seasoning, salt, and pepper. Place in the oven and broil for 10 minutes or until the salmon flakes easily with a fork.

2. While the salmon is cooking, in a mixing bowl combine the ingredients for the topping.

3. Remove the salmon from the oven and serve topped with the tomato topping.

Makes 6 servings | Per serving: Calories: 344, Fat: 22g, Total CARBS: 5g, Fiber: 1g, Protein: 32g

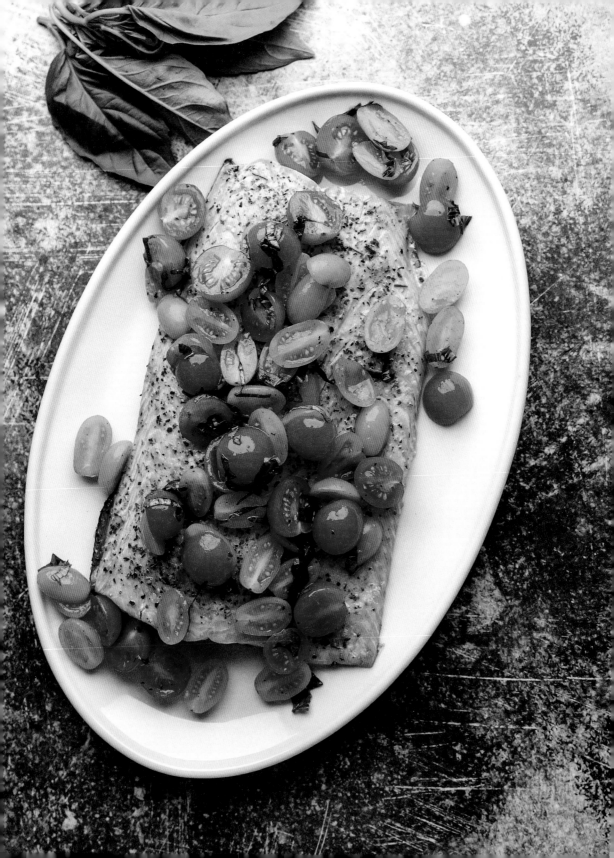

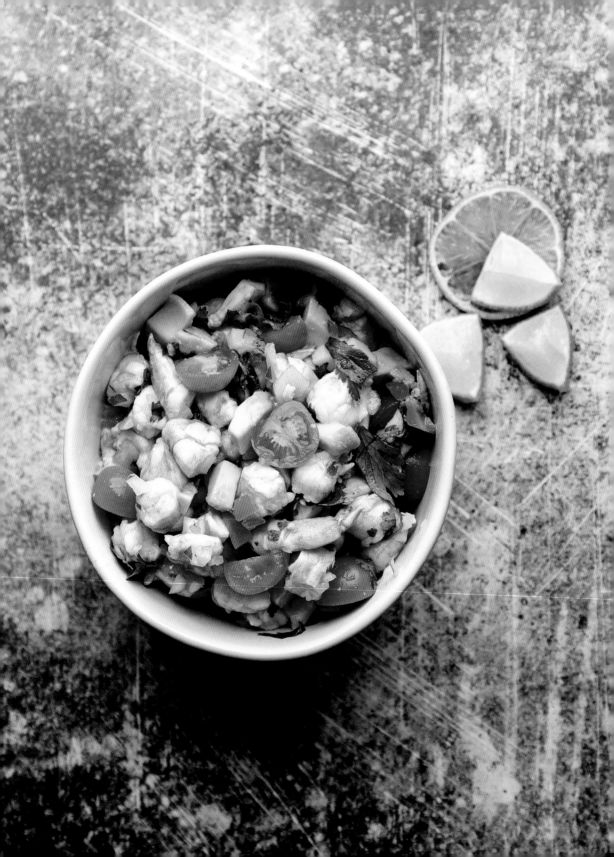

SHRIMP CEVICHE

Traditionally, ceviche is made with raw fish, and the acid from the citrus juice "cooks" it. I have found that using pre-cooked shrimp works just as well and gives me a little peace of mind. This dish is on the lighter side and goes perfectly wrapped in butter lettuce leaves.

Prep Time: 40 minutes | Total Time: 40 minutes

1 pound peeled and deveined pre-cooked shrimp

⅓ cup fresh lime juice

2 tablespoons avocado oil

⅓ cup finely diced red onion

¼ cup finely diced red bell pepper

¼ cup chopped cilantro

¼ teaspoon kosher salt

2 whole avocados, diced

10 cherry tomatoes, sliced in half lengthwise

8 butter lettuce leaves (optional)

Chop the cooked shrimp into 1-inch pieces and add to a large mixing bowl. Combine with the rest of the ingredients and let marinate for at least 30 minutes. Serve in butter lettuce leaves.

Makes 4 servings | Per serving: Calories: 332, Fat: 20g, Total CARBS: 11g, Fiber: 6g, Protein: 28g

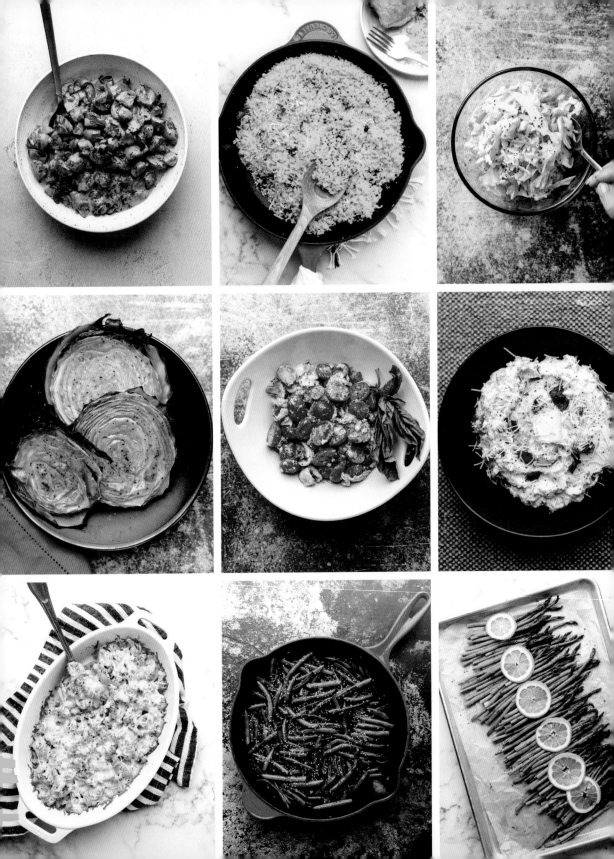

SIDE DISHES

LEMON ROASTED ASPARAGUS

This is the perfect spring side dish when you're looking for something quick and easy. Choose asparagus with tips that are tightly closed and stalks that are firm.

Prep Time: 5 minutes | Cook Time: 13 minutes | Total Time: 18 minutes

2 bunches asparagus, woody
    ends removed

4 tablespoons butter, melted

½ teaspoon kosher salt

¼ teaspoon black pepper

Juice of 1 lemon

1 lemon, sliced

1. Preheat the oven to 400°F and line a baking sheet with parchment paper.

2. Spread the asparagus across the center, drizzle with the melted butter, and season with salt and pepper. Pour the lemon juice over the top of the asparagus and, finally, lay the lemon slices across the top.

3. Bake for 10–13 minutes or until the asparagus is fork tender.

Makes 4 servings | Per serving: Calories: 130, Fat: 12g, Total CARBS: 7g, Fiber: 3g, Protein: 3g

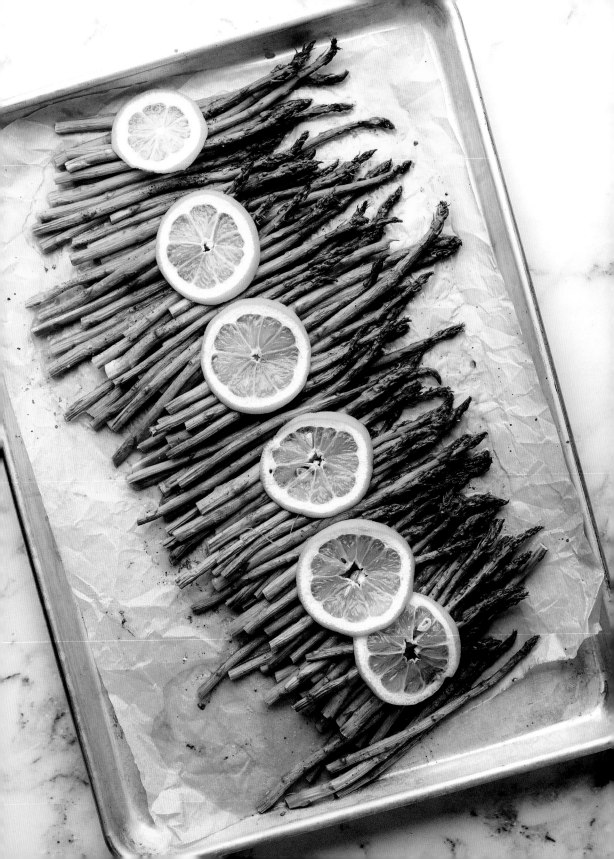

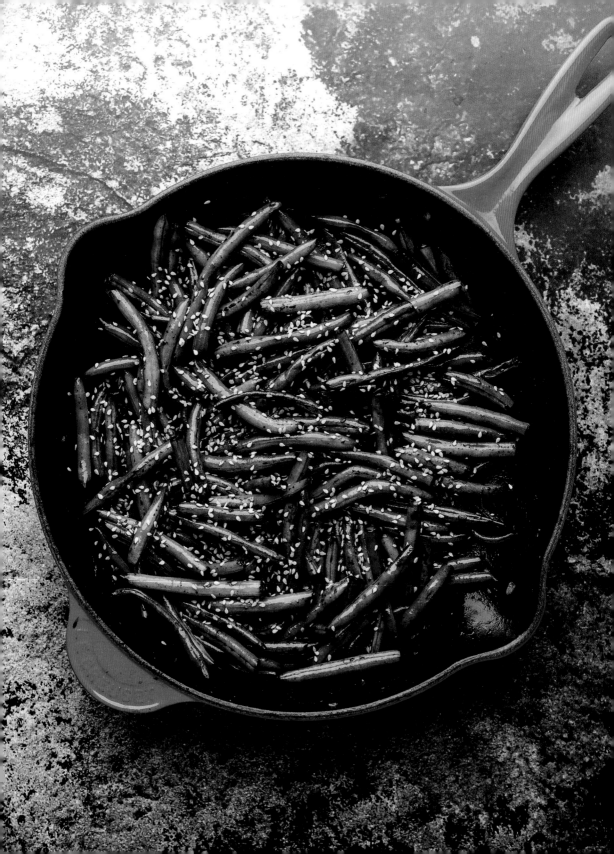

SESAME GARLIC GREEN BEANS

I was raised on canned green beans, but nothing beats fresh! The East Asian–inspired flavors in these beans make them just amazing alongside your favorite grilled protein and teriyaki sauce (see my keto-friendly Teriyaki Sauce on page 265). If you avoid gluten, choose tamari or coconut aminos instead of soy sauce.

Prep Time: 5 minutes | Cook Time: 10 minutes | Total Time: 15 minutes

1 pound fresh green beans, ends trimmed

2 tablespoons soy sauce, tamari, or coconut aminos

½ tablespoon sesame oil

½ tablespoon minced garlic

½ tablespoon white sesame seeds

1. In a large skillet over medium-high heat, stir together the green beans, soy sauce, and sesame oil. Stir frequently until beans are tender but still crisp, about 5 minutes. Stir in the minced garlic and cook for 1 minute more until fragrant.

2. Remove from the heat and stir in the sesame seeds.

Makes 4 servings | Per serving: Calories: 73, Fat: 3g, Total CARBS: 9g, Fiber: 3g, Protein: 4g

CREAMY GARLIC MUSHROOMS

Mushrooms are the perfect keto-friendly vegetable at only 5 net carbs per ½ pound. That's a lot of mushrooms! The rich and creamy sauce in this recipe pairs perfectly with the mushrooms and makes this an indulgent side that's especially nice for a dinner party or family gathering.

Prep Time: 5 minutes | Cook Time: 20 minutes | Total Time: 25 minutes

1 tablespoon butter

1 tablespoon avocado oil

2 pounds mushrooms, stalks trimmed, quartered

½ teaspoon kosher salt

¼ teaspoon pepper

6 garlic cloves, minced

½ teaspoon dried thyme

1 cup heavy cream

Chopped fresh parsley, for garnish (optional)

1. Heat the butter and avocado oil in a large skillet over medium-high heat. Add the mushrooms, salt, and pepper. Let cook for 5 minutes, stirring occasionally, until the mushrooms are soft. Stir in the garlic and thyme and cook for 1 minute more until fragrant.

2. Stir in the heavy cream, reduce the heat to medium-low, and let simmer for 20 minutes, until the liquid is reduced and thickened. Transfer the mushrooms and sauce to a serving bowl and garnish with chopped fresh parsley if desired.

Makes 6 servings | Per serving: Calories: 214, Fat: 21g, Total CARBS: 7g, Fiber: 2g, Protein: 6g

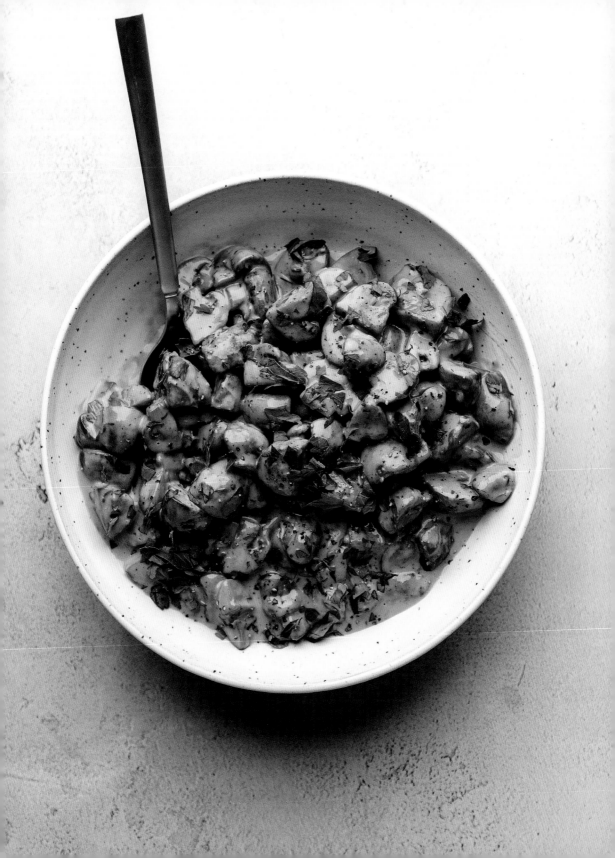

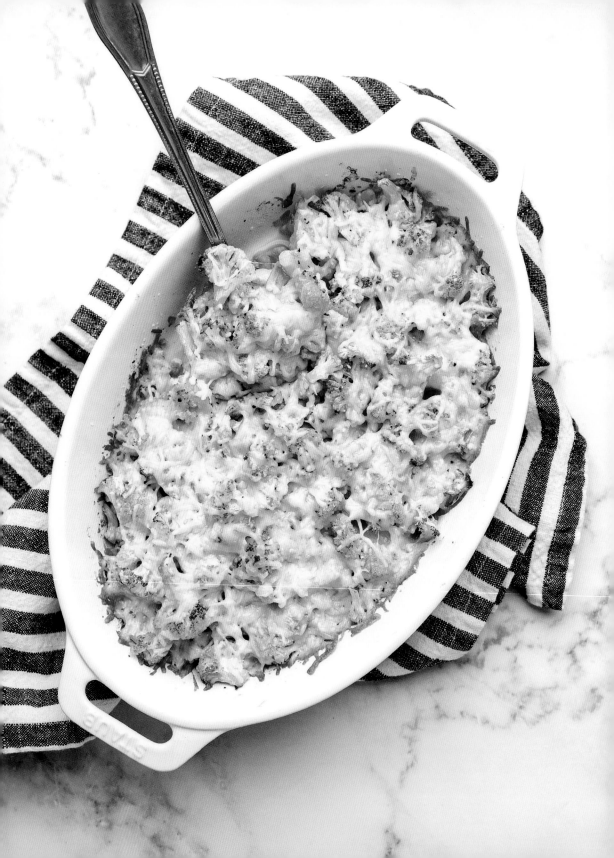

CHEESY BAKED CAULIFLOWER

This is my go-to cauliflower recipe because it is so easy and tastes amazing! This recipe works with any shredded cheese you like, if you prefer others to Parmesan (or use a blend!). I have used cheddar and Monterey jack with great results.

Prep Time: 10 minutes | Cook Time: 30 minutes | Total Time: 40 minutes

1 large head of cauliflower, chopped into small florets

3 tablespoons avocado oil

Salt and freshly ground black pepper

1 cup shredded Parmesan cheese

1. Preheat the oven to 400°F and grease a 9 × 13–inch baking dish.

2. Pour the cauliflower into the baking dish and drizzle with the oil. Season with salt and pepper.

3. Bake for 30 minutes until the cauliflower starts to brown and is fork tender.

4. Remove from the oven, sprinkle with the Parmesan cheese, and bake for an additional 5–8 minutes, until the cheese is melted and starts to brown.

Makes 6 servings | Per serving: Calories: 155, Fat: 11g, Protein: 7g, Total CARBS: 7g, Fiber: 2g

BACON AND BRUSSELS SPROUT BAKE

Brussels sprouts with bacon are a classic keto side dish. Add Swiss cheese and we take it over the top! The frozen Brussels sprouts are key in this recipe because they don't need as much time to cook. If you would like to use fresh Brussels sprouts, trim the ends, slice in half lengthwise, and simmer in a pot of boiling water for five minutes, then drain.

Prep Time: 10 minutes | Cook Time: 40 minutes | Total Time: 50 minutes

6 slices thick-cut bacon, diced

½ white onion, sliced thin

20 ounces frozen Brussels sprouts, thawed and halved

1½ cups shredded Swiss cheese

½ cup heavy cream

½ teaspoon kosher salt

¼ teaspoon pepper

1. Preheat the oven to 400°F and spray an 8 × 11–inch casserole dish with cooking spray.

2. Heat a large skillet over medium-high heat. Cook the bacon and the onion in the skillet until the bacon is crispy and the onion is soft, about 10 minutes. Drain on a plate lined with paper towels.

3. In a large mixing bowl combine the Brussels sprouts, Swiss cheese, cream, salt, pepper, and the bacon and onions. Pour the mixture into the casserole dish and bake for 30 minutes or until the sprouts are tender.

Makes 8 servings | Per serving: Calories: 264, Fat: 18g, Total CARBS: 14g, Fiber: 5g, Protein: 13g

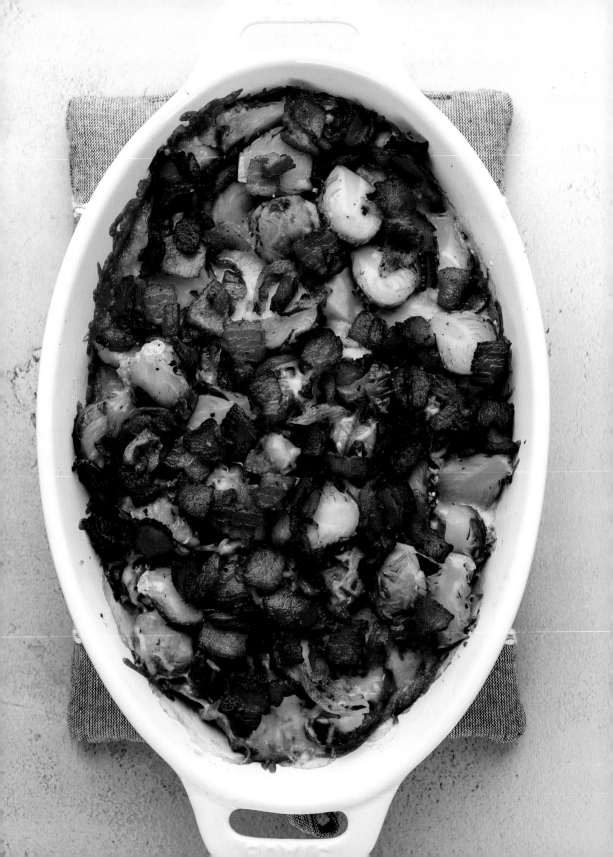

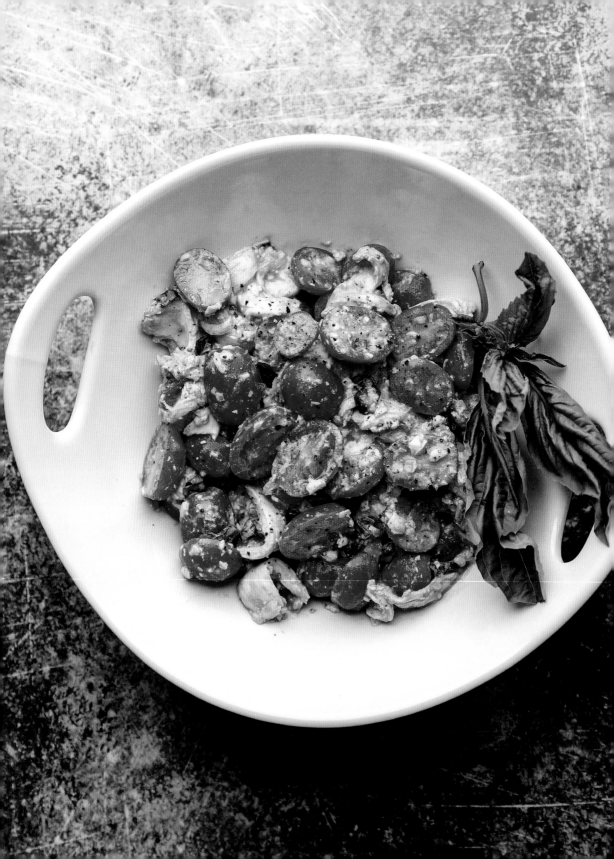

TOMATO AND BURRATA SALAD

Burrata is the cheese buzzword of the moment and for good reason. It is rich and creamy and makes a lovely flavor contrast to bright tomatoes. If you are having trouble finding burrata, you can substitute fresh mozzarella in this recipe.

Prep Time: 10 minutes | Total Time: 10 minutes

10 ounces grape tomatoes, halved

8 ounces burrata cheese, torn into 1-inch chunks

3 garlic cloves, minced

2 tablespoons balsamic vinegar

1 tablespoon olive oil

4 basil leaves, chopped

½ teaspoon kosher salt

¼ teaspoon pepper

Combine all ingredients in a large mixing bowl. Toss to combine and evenly coat the tomatoes and cheese with the flavorings. Serve immediately.

Makes 4 servings | Per serving: Calories: 214, Fat: 18g, Total CARBS: 7g, Fiber: 2g, Protein: 7g

ROASTED CABBAGE STEAKS

Looking for a new and exciting way to cook your veggies? These baked cabbage "steaks"—tender inside, browned and crispy outside—are an easy and tasty way to get an extra serving of vegetables.

Prep Time: 5 minutes | Cook Time: 40 minutes | Total Time: 45 minutes

¼ cup avocado oil

1 teaspoon garlic powder

1 teaspoon kosher salt

¼ teaspoon black pepper

1 small head of green cabbage, tough outer leaves and core removed (yield 1.5 pounds)

1. Preheat the oven to 400°F and line a large rimmed baking sheet with parchment paper.

2. In a small mixing bowl combine the avocado oil, garlic powder, salt, and pepper.

3. Cut the cabbage into 1-inch-thick slices and place them in a single layer on the baking sheet. Use a basting brush to brush the tops of the cabbage steaks with the avocado oil mixture. Bake the cabbage for 30–40 minutes or until the centers are fork tender and the outsides are crispy.

Makes 4 servings | Per serving: Calories: 177, Fat: 14g, Total CARBS: 11g, Fiber: 4g, Protein: 2g

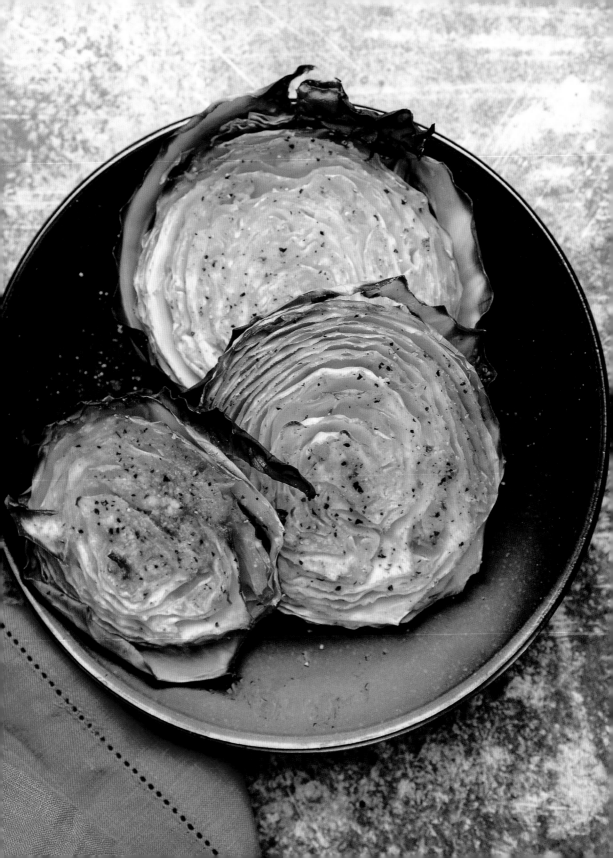

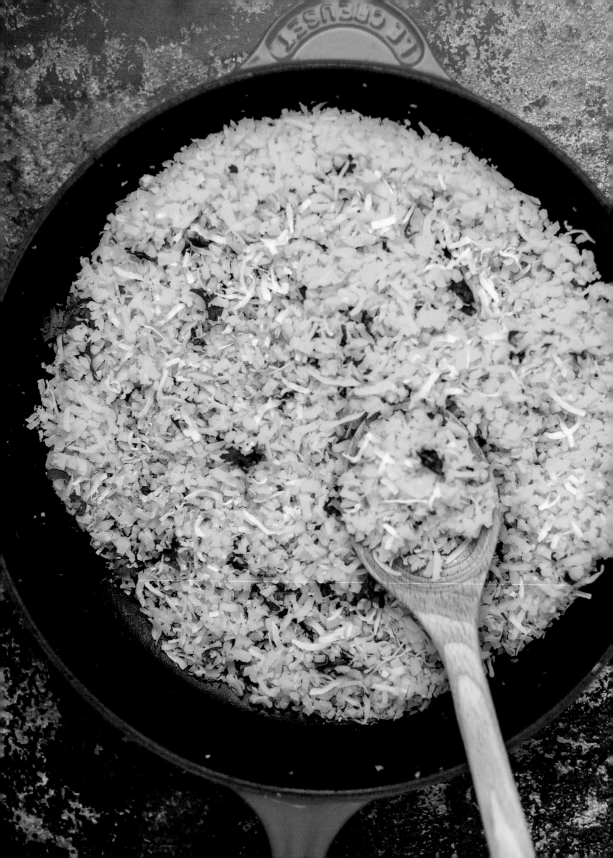

TURMERIC CAULIFLOWER RICE WITH COCONUT

This is such a flavorful side dish—a bright and unusual take on cauliflower rice. The shredded coconut adds a lovely texture.

Prep Time: 10 minutes | Cook Time: 5 minutes | Total Time: 15 minutes

1 medium head of cauliflower or 16 ounces frozen cauliflower rice

2 tablespoons coconut oil

2 garlic cloves, minced

½ teaspoon ground turmeric

Salt to taste

¼ cup unsweetened shredded coconut

¼ cup chopped fresh cilantro

1. Chop the cauliflower into small pieces (including the core) and pulse in the food processor until it resembles rice. Skip this step if you're using frozen cauliflower rice.

2. Heat the coconut oil in a large skillet over medium heat. Stir in the cauliflower rice, garlic, and turmeric, and season with salt. Sauté, stirring occasionally, for about 5 minutes or until the cauliflower is tender and starting to brown.

3. Stir in the shredded coconut and cilantro and cook for 1 minute more.

Makes 4 servings | Per serving: Calories: 123, Fat: 10g, Total CARBS: 7g, Fiber: 4g, Protein: 3g

GRUYÈRE MASHED CAULIFLOWER

Gruyère is a firm, pale Swiss cheese with a rich and slightly nutty flavor. If you prefer to use another variety of Swiss (or even a cheddar) in this delicious mash, please do! This cheesy mashed cauliflower reminds me of the French dish *pommes aligot*, which are mashed potatoes with lots and lots of melted cheese. Enjoy!

Prep Time: 10 minutes | Cook Time: 10 minutes | Total Time: 20 minutes

1 large head cauliflower, cut into small florets (approximately 1.5 pounds)

1 cup heavy cream

2 cups grated Gruyère cheese

½ teaspoon kosher salt

½ teaspoon pepper

¼ teaspoon ground nutmeg

4 slices thick bacon, cooked and crumbled

1. Bring a large pot of salted water to a boil. Boil the cauliflower florets for 5 minutes or until fork tender. Drain and set aside.

2. In a small saucepan bring the heavy cream to a boil. Remove from the heat and add the cheese, salt, pepper, and nutmeg. Stir well to melt the cheese into the cream.

3. In a blender, blend the cauliflower with the cheese sauce until smooth and creamy. Add the bacon and pulse a few times to incorporate. Scrape from the blender to a large serving bowl.

Makes 6 servings | Per serving: Calories: 342, Fat: 30g, Total CARBS: 7g, Fiber: 3g, Protein: 16g

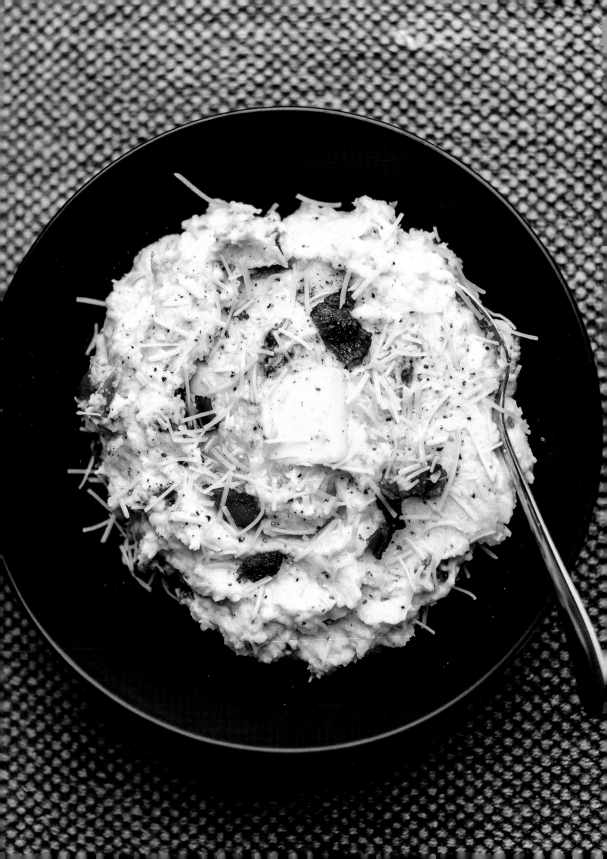

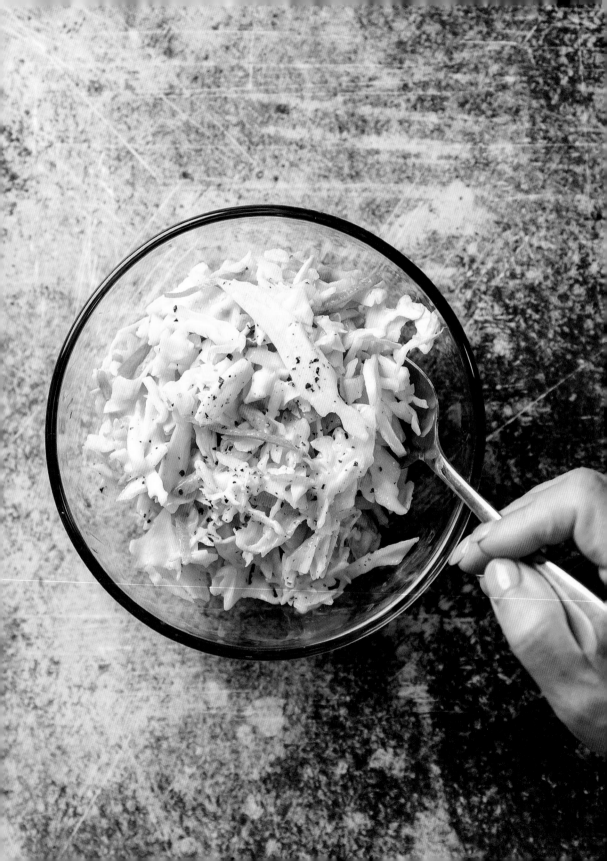

CRUNCHY COLESLAW

Store-bought coleslaw or coleslaw in restaurants usually contains sugar—so close to keto-friendly, yet so far! With a simple swap, we take this dish from no to yes.

Prep Time: 5 minutes | Total Time: 5 minutes

16 ounces shredded cabbage or bagged slaw mix

½ cup mayonnaise

1 tablespoon granulated sweetener

2½ tablespoons apple cider vinegar

Kosher salt and pepper to taste

Combine all ingredients in a large mixing bowl and season with salt and pepper. Taste the slaw and adjust the flavors to your liking, adding more vinegar, salt, or pepper as needed.

Makes 6 servings | Per serving: Calories: 144, Fat: 14g, Total CARBS: 4g, Fiber: 2g, Protein:1g

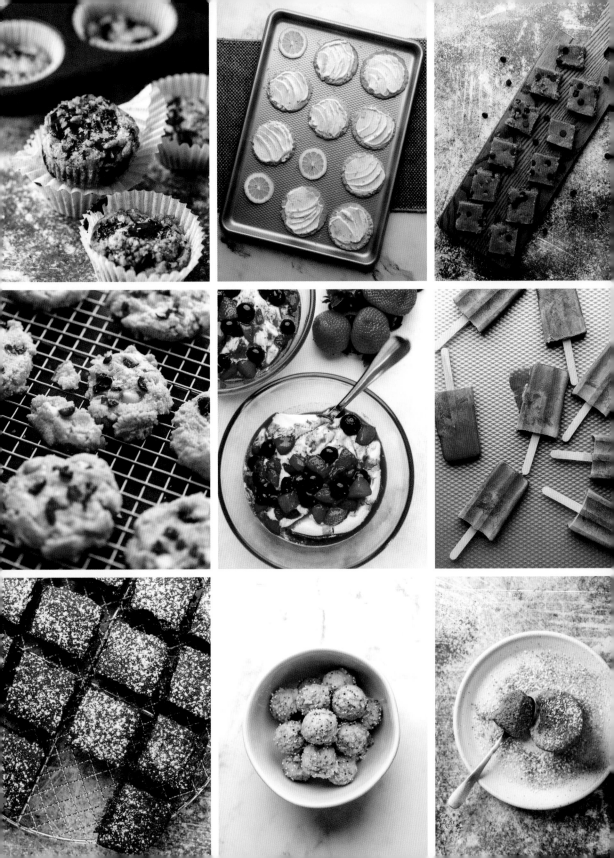

DESSERTS

BROWNED BUTTER CHOCOLATE CHUNK COOKIE CUPS

The browned butter cannot be skipped in this recipe. It adds a little time, but the rich flavor it adds to the final recipe is incredible!

Prep Time: 10 minutes | Cook Time: 15 minutes | Total Time: 25 minutes

⅓ cup butter

1½ cups almond flour

½ cup granulated sweetener

½ teaspoon baking soda

¼ teaspoon kosher salt

1 large egg

1 teaspoon vanilla extract

6 ounces 86 percent cacao dark chocolate bar, chopped

Makes 12 cookie cups, 1 per serving | Per serving: Calories: 213, Fat: 21g, Total CARBS: 8g, Fiber: 3g, Protein: 4g

1. Brown the butter: In a small saucepan over medium heat, melt the butter and continue to cook, stirring frequently. The butter will begin to foam and sizzle—keep stirring. When the milk solids in the butter begin to brown and the butter takes on a nutty aroma, remove from the heat and set aside.

2. Preheat the oven to 350°F. Line a 12-cup muffin pan with liners and spray the inside of the liners with cooking spray.

3. Combine the almond flour, sweetener, baking soda, and salt in a large mixing bowl and stir until well combined. Stir in the browned butter, egg, and vanilla until well combined. Finally, fold in the chopped chocolate.

4. Divide the batter evenly within the prepared muffin pan. Flatten out the tops with the back of a spoon. Bake for 15–17 minutes, until the edges begin to brown and a toothpick inserted in the center comes out clean. Let cool in the pan for 10 minutes and then remove to a wire rack to cool completely.

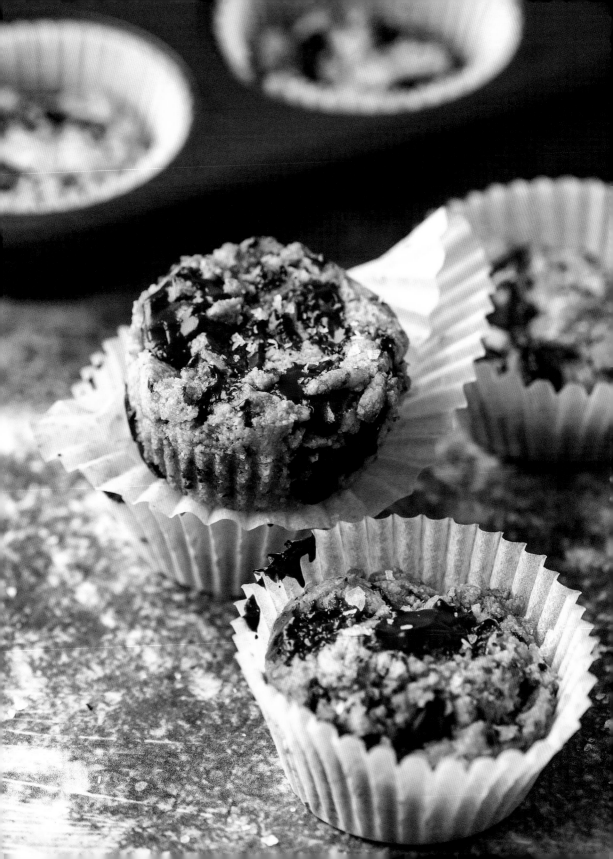

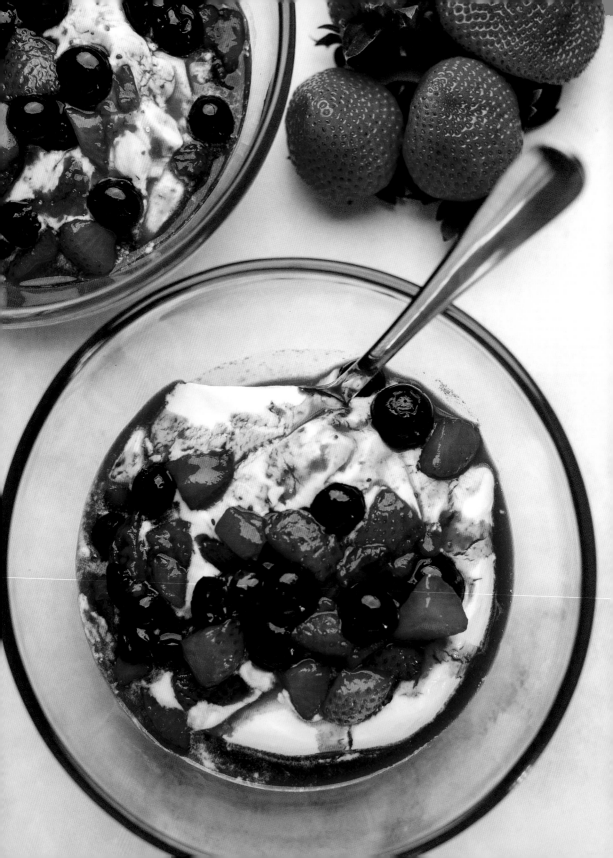

BERRY YOGURT PARFAIT

By combining the whipped heavy cream with Greek yogurt, we make this an incredibly rich but still light and amazing keto-friendly dessert.

Prep Time: 5 minutes | Cook Time: 8 minutes | Total Time: 13 minutes

½ cup blueberries

½ cup strawberries, chopped

⅓ cup plus 1 tablespoon granulated sweetener, divided

¾ cup heavy cream

1 tablespoon vanilla extract

1½ cups unsweetened fat-free Greek yogurt

1. In a small saucepan over medium heat, combine the berries with 1 tablespoon of sweetener. Cook for 5–8 minutes, until the berries release their juices. Remove from the heat and set aside.

2. In a medium-sized mixing bowl beat the heavy cream, vanilla, and ⅓ cup sweetener until stiff peaks form. Fold in the Greek yogurt. Divide the mixture among 4 bowls and top with the berries.

Makes 4 servings | Per serving: Calories: 214, Fat: 18g, Total CARBS: 7g, Fiber: 1g, Protein: 8g

CHOCOLATE SNACK CAKE

This is such a great snack to have on hand, especially when you're first starting out with keto, because it is super easy to make and it fulfills that sweet chocolate craving. Store in an airtight container in the refrigerator for up to one week.

Prep Time: 5 minutes | Cook Time: 30 minutes | Total Time: 35 minutes

2½ cups almond flour

½ cup cocoa powder

⅔ cup granulated sweetener

1 teaspoon baking soda

½ teaspoon kosher salt

8 ounces unsweetened fat-free Greek yogurt

4 large eggs, beaten

2 teaspoons vanilla extract

Powdered sweetener, for garnish

1. Preheat the oven to 350°F and spray a 9 × 9–inch ceramic baking pan with cooking spray.

2. In a large mixing bowl combine the almond flour, cocoa powder, granulated sweetener, baking soda, and salt until well combined. Stir in the Greek yogurt, eggs, and vanilla.

3. Pour the batter into the baking pan and bake for 35 minutes or until a toothpick inserted into the center comes out clean. Let cool for 10 minutes and then cut into 16 squares. Sprinkle powdered sweetener on top for garnish.

Note: This recipe specifies a ceramic baking dish. If you use a metal pan, the outside of the cake may overbake before the inside is done. Watch carefully!

Makes 16 servings | Per serving: Calories: 132, Fat: 9g, Total CARBS: 4g, Fiber: 3g, Protein: 6g

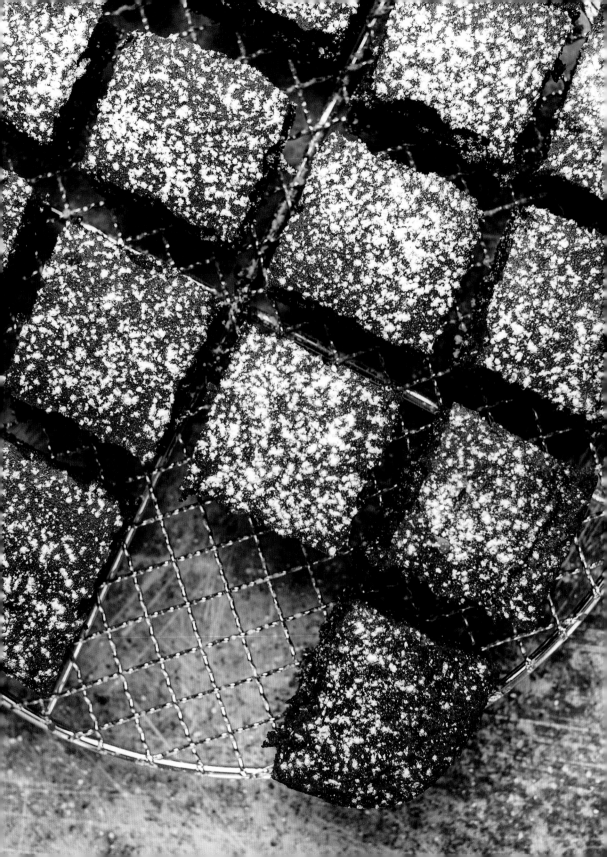

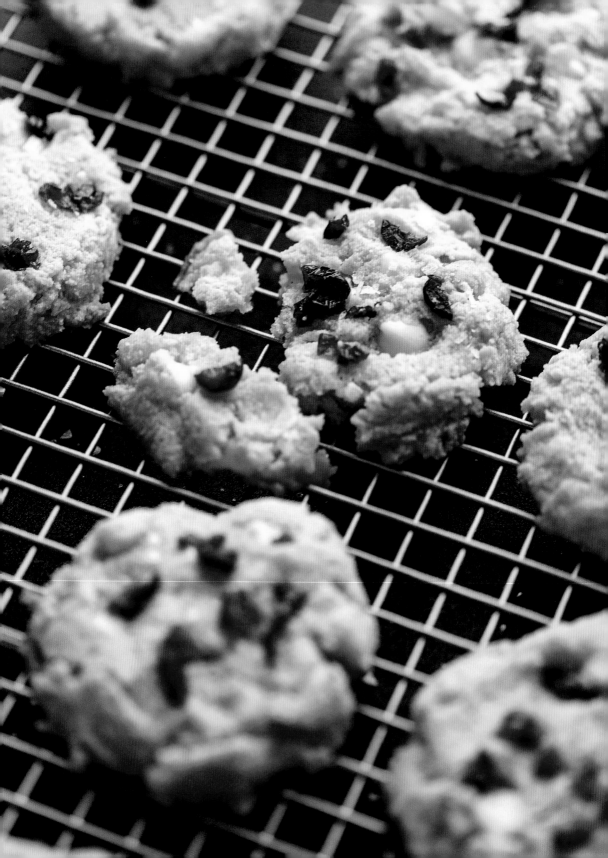

WHITE CHOCOLATE MACADAMIA NUT COOKIES WITH CRANBERRIES

The combination of sweet white chocolate and tart cranberries in these cookies is amazing! Look for a dried cranberry that has no added sugar or fruit juices. If your grocery store doesn't carry them, try online.

Prep Time: 10 minutes | Cook Time: 15 minutes | Total Time: 25 minutes

3 cups almond flour

⅔ cup granulated sweetener

½ teaspoon baking soda

½ teaspoon kosher salt

2 eggs, beaten

¾ cup butter, softened

2 teaspoons vanilla extract

9 ounces sugar-free white chocolate chips (I like Lily's brand)

½ cup chopped macadamia nuts

¼ cup dried cranberries

1. Preheat the oven to 350°F and line 2 rimmed baking sheets with parchment paper.

2. In a large mixing bowl combine the almond flour, sweetener, baking soda, and salt until well combined. Use an electric mixer to mix in the eggs, butter, and vanilla extract. Now fold in the chocolate chips and macadamia nuts.

3. Divide the batter into 24 rounds evenly spaced on the 2 baking sheets. Press the dried cranberries on top. Bake in the oven for 15 minutes, rotating baking sheets halfway through, or until the cookies are set and start to brown around the edges.

4. Remove from the oven and let cool completely. Store in an airtight container for up to 1 week.

Makes 24 cookies; 1 per serving | Per serving: Calories: 207, Fat: 19g, Total CARBS: 6g, Fiber: 2g, Protein: 5g

NO-BAKE CHOCOLATE CHIP PROTEIN BITES

Using protein powder in baked goods and desserts is a great way to boost your overall protein intake. My favorite kind is Premier Protein's Vanilla Milkshake Protein Powder, but if the brand isn't available to you, look for one that's low in carbs. These are the perfect little sweet bite!

Prep Time: 10 minutes | Set Time: 2 hours | Total Time: 2 hours 10 minutes

1½ cups almond flour

⅓ cup vanilla protein powder

3 tablespoons granulated sweetener

¼ teaspoon kosher salt

½ cup creamy sugar-free almond butter

¼ cup half-and-half

1 teaspoon vanilla extract

½ cup sugar-free chocolate chips

1. In a large mixing bowl, combine the almond flour, protein powder, sweetener, and salt. Mix in the almond butter, half-and-half, vanilla, and chocolate chips until well combined. The batter will be very thick, so you may need to mix with your hands.

2. Transfer the mixture into an 8 × 8–inch baking dish and press into a single layer with your hands. Refrigerate for 2 hours or until completely set. Cut into 16 squares.

Makes 16 protein bites; 1 per serving | Per serving: Calories: 119, Fat: 10g, Total CARBS: 3g, Fiber: 2g, Protein: 6g

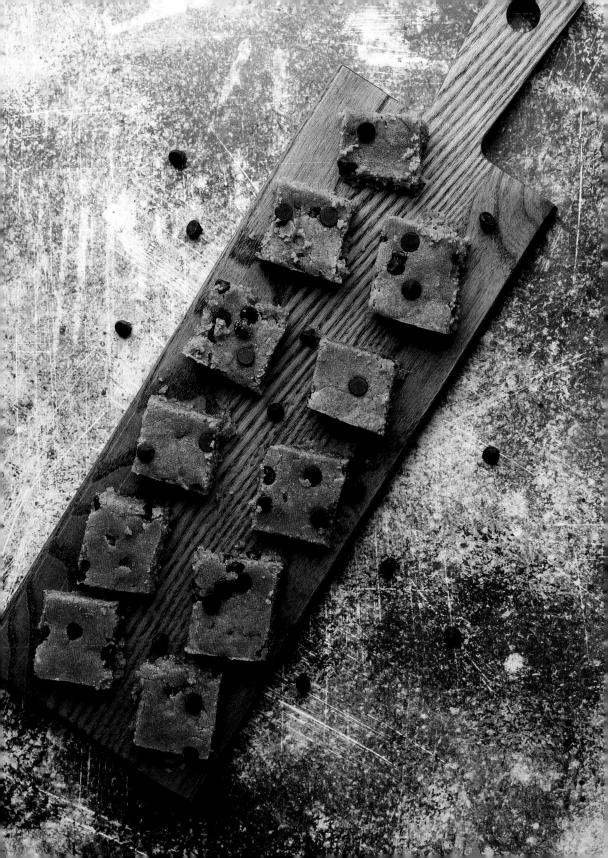

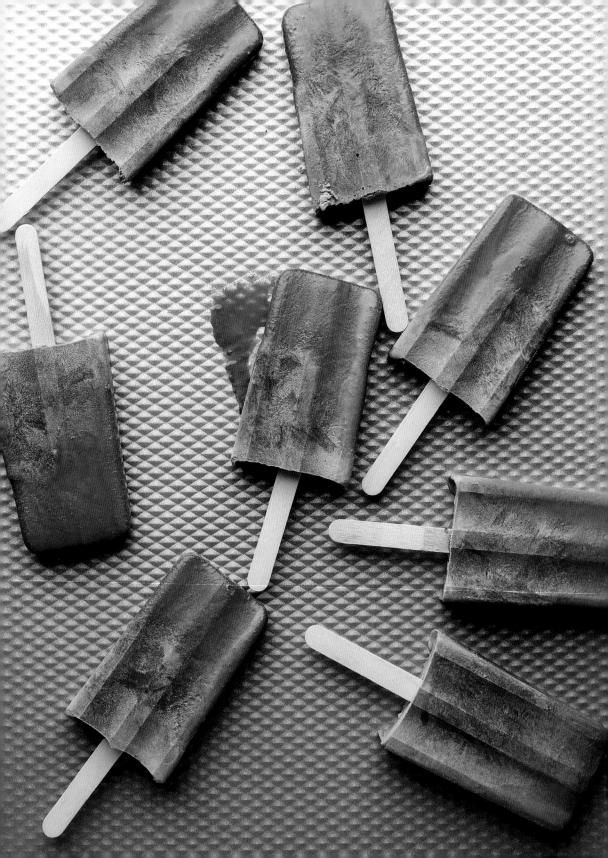

FUDGE POPS

These will be a hit not just with kids, but adults, too! Honestly, you will probably want to make a double batch every time you make these because they are so good! My trick to making these just like the store-bought kind is to partially freeze the pops before you put the sticks in the molds. That way, the sticks won't sink all the way to the tops of the pops.

Prep Time: 15 minutes | Cook Time: 5 minutes | Set Time: 4 hours | Total Time: 4 hours, 20 minutes

2 cups half-and-half

½ cup granulated sweetener

⅓ cup cocoa powder

1 teaspoon vanilla extract

Pinch of salt

1. Whisk together all ingredients in a small saucepan over medium heat. Whisk continuously until the cocoa powder fully dissolves, about 5 minutes. Let cool for 10 minutes.

2. Once mixture is cooled, pour evenly into an ice pop mold. This should make about 8 fudge pops depending on the size of your mold.

3. Place the mold into the freezer for about 2 hours until the pops are thick and partially frozen. Take the mold out of the freezer and carefully insert wooden or plastic treat sticks into the mold. Place back into the freezer for another 2 hours or until completely frozen.

Makes about 8 fudge pops; 1 per serving | Per serving: Calories: 108, Fat: 7g, Total CARBS: 5g, Fiber: 1g, Protein: 2g

BIRTHDAY CAKE FAT BOMBS

My daughter loves the birthday cake pops from a popular coffee chain so I thought I would re-create a keto version that she might like just as well. These are just as good (and only 2g carbs each)!

Prep Time: 10 minutes | Set Time: 20 minutes | Total Time: 30 minutes

1 cup almond flour

3 tablespoons granulated sweetener

4 ounces cream cheese, softened

1 teaspoon vanilla extract

1 tablespoon sprinkles plus more for garnish

Pinch of salt

1. In a medium-sized mixing bowl combine all the ingredients until well mixed.

2. Use a 1-tablespoon cookie scoop to evenly scoop the batter into 18 fat bombs. Place them on a plate or rimmed baking sheet. Top with extra sprinkles for garnish.

3. Refrigerate for 20 minutes to set. Keep refrigerated until ready to serve; fat bombs will keep chilled for up to 1 week.

Makes 18 fat bombs; 1 per serving | Per serving: Calories: 64, Fat: 6g, Total CARBS: 2g, Fiber: 1g, Protein: 1g

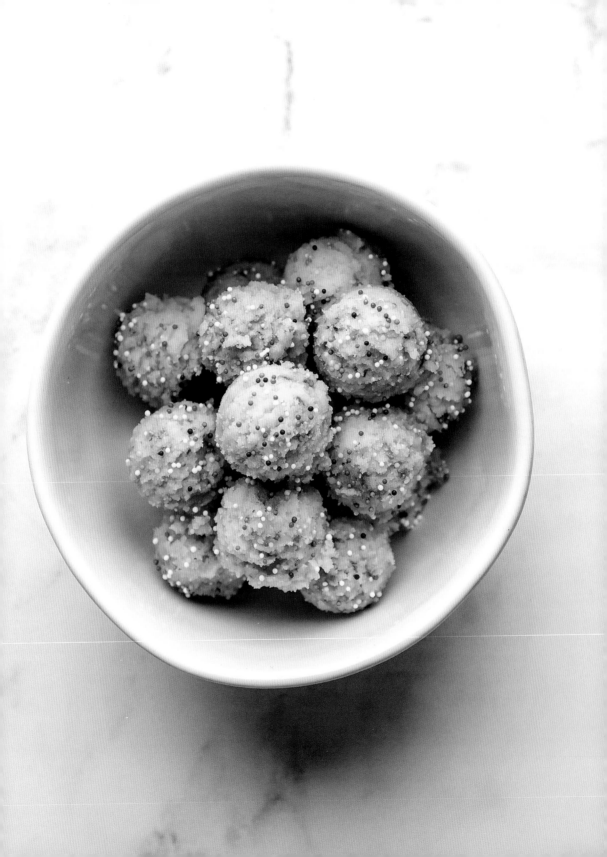

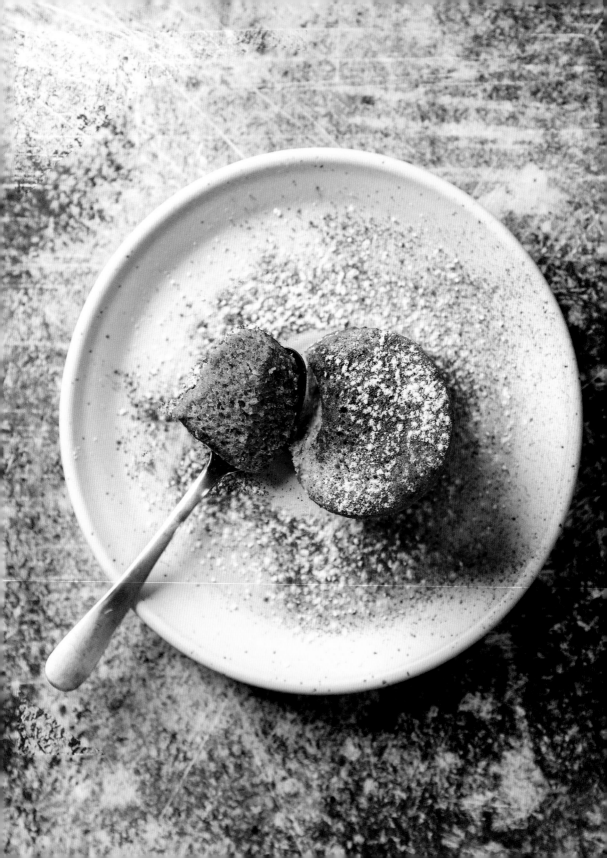

SNICKERDOODLE MUG CAKE

Quick and easy mug cakes give me life on the keto diet when I want something sweet. On my blog, *Low Carb with Jennifer*, I've offered recipes for chocolate, vanilla, and peanut butter mug cakes. Let me just tell you, this snickerdoodle flavor is by far my favorite! It is a delicious dense cake that tastes just like an amazing snickerdoodle cookie.

Prep Time: 5 minutes | Cook Time: 1 minute, 30 seconds | Total Time: 6 minutes, 30 seconds

1 tablespoon butter

3 tablespoons almond flour

2 tablespoons granulated sweetener

1 large egg, beaten

½ teaspoon baking powder

½ teaspoon cinnamon, plus extra for garnish

Splash of vanilla extract

Powdered sweetener, for garnish (optional)

1. In a microwave-safe mug or ramekin, microwave the butter for 10 seconds to melt it. Swirl the butter around the inside of the mug to grease the sides. (Leave any remaining melted butter in the mug—it's part of the batter, too!)

2. Add the almond flour, sweetener, egg, baking powder, cinnamon, and vanilla. Whisk well until combined.

3. Microwave for 60 seconds. Let stand in the microwave for 1 minute before removing. If you like, invert the cake onto a plate or enjoy it right in the mug. Sprinkle with extra cinnamon and powdered sweetener for a garnish, if desired.

Makes 1 mug cake; 1 per serving | Per serving: Calories: 304, Fat: 28g, Total CARBS: 5g, Fiber: 3g, Protein: 11g

ICED LEMON COOKIES

These melt-in-your-mouth lemon cookies with lemon cream cheese icing are the perfect easy treat for a picnic. The lemon flavor is so refreshing, especially with fresh-squeezed lemon juice!

Prep Time: 10 minutes | Cook Time: 12 minutes | Total Time: 22 minutes

1½ cups almond flour

⅓ cup powdered sweetener

¼ teaspoon baking soda

Pinch of kosher salt

Zest of 1 lemon

½ cup softened butter

1 teaspoon vanilla extract

Lemon Cream Cheese Icing

⅓ cup powdered sweetener

2 ounces softened cream cheese

1 tablespoon fresh-squeezed lemon juice

½ teaspoon vanilla extract

1. Preheat the oven to 350°F and line a cookie sheet with parchment paper or a silicone baking mat.

2. In a large mixing bowl combine the almond flour, powdered sweetener, baking soda, salt, and lemon zest. Add the softened butter and vanilla extract and use an electric mixer to combine until all of the almond flour is mixed into the butter.

3. Use a 2-tablespoon cookie scoop or a spoon to divide the batter into 9 cookies and flatten out the tops. Bake for 12 minutes or until the edges turn golden brown. Let cool for 10 minutes on the baking sheet before icing.

4. While the cookies are baking, make the icing. Combine all icing ingredients in a medium-sized mixing bowl and beat with a hand mixer until fully combined.

5. Spread the icing over each cookie before serving.

Makes 9 cookies; 1 per serving | Per serving: Calories: 300, Fat: 22g, Total CARBS: 4g, Fiber: 2g, Protein: 5g

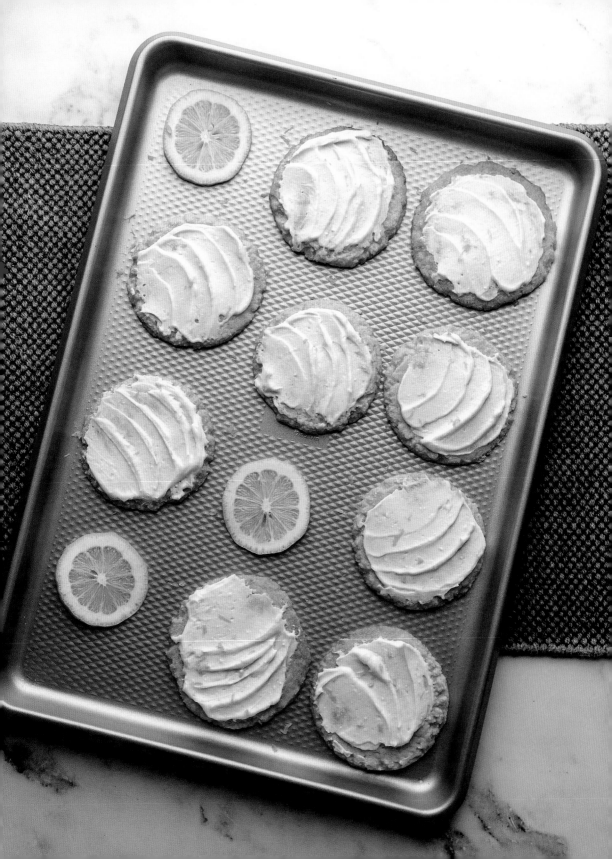

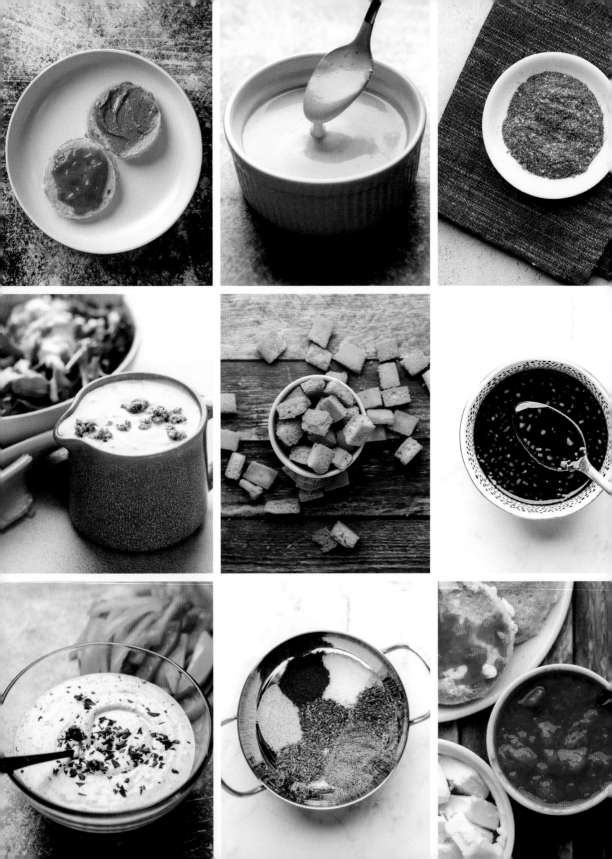

BASICS

BBQ DRY RUB

This dry rub is the perfect sweet and salty seasoning for any time you are ready to throw some meat on the grill. I love to use this for pork, such as for my Pulled Pork Sandwiches (page 191), but it works perfectly for chicken as well.

Prep Time: 10 minutes | Total Time: 10 minutes

¼ cup brown sugar sweetener

1 tablespoon kosher salt

1 tablespoon chili powder

2 teaspoons ground black pepper

2 teaspoons smoked paprika

2 teaspoons garlic powder

2 teaspoons onion powder

1 teaspoon ground mustard

1 teaspoon turmeric

Makes 9 tablespoons;
1 tablespoon per serving | Per
serving: Calories: 12, Fat: 0g,
Total CARBS: 2g, Protein: 1g,
Fiber: 1g

Combine all ingredients in a small mixing bowl. Store in an airtight container for up to 1 month.

Note: The ingredients will cake together if left to sit. This is from the lack of an anti-caking agent. Simply shake the jar before each use and you're good to go.

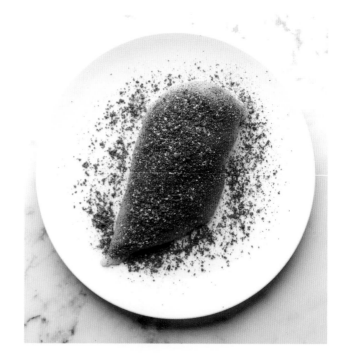

TACO SEASONING

Taco seasoning mixes are so convenient, but many store-bought brands are full of things like cornstarch, maltodextrin, and sugar. This one is clean as a whistle and packed with flavor.

Prep Time: 5 minutes | Total Time: 5 minutes

1½ teaspoons kosher salt

1½ teaspoons cumin

½ teaspoon onion powder

½ teaspoon garlic powder

½ teaspoon chili powder

½ teaspoon smoked paprika

Makes 5 teaspoons;
1¼ teaspoons per serving | Per serving: Calories: 6, Fat: 0g, Total CARBS: 1g, Fiber: 0g, Protein: 0g

Combine all ingredients in a small mixing bowl. Store in an airtight container for up to 1 month. Use 2 tablespoons per 1 pound of ground meat.

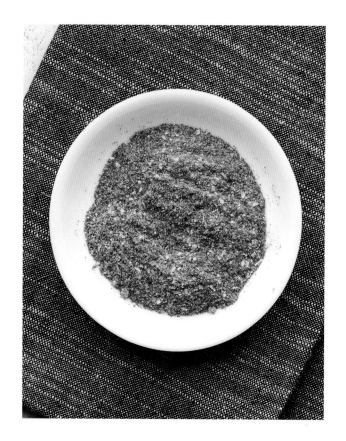

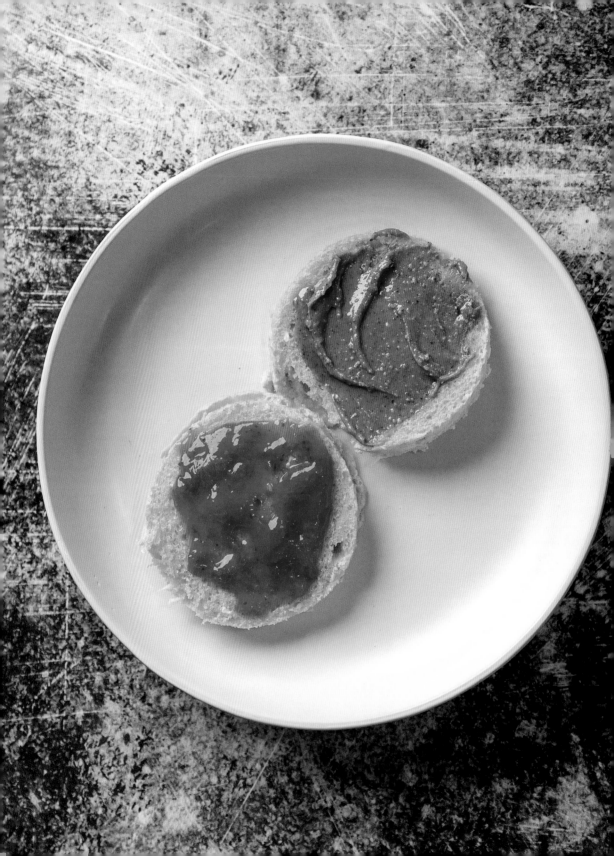

MICROWAVE BREAD

Bread on keto can be kind of tricky unless you have this recipe in your back pocket!
I love to toast it up on the stove (toasting it gives it a wonderful texture!) and apply
a generous serving of butter or sugar-free jam and almond butter. This can also
be used for sandwiches or hamburger buns! If you would prefer to bake this in the
oven, use an oven-safe container and bake at 350°F for eight to ten minutes.

Prep Time: 5 minutes | Cook Time: 2 minutes | Total Time: 7 minutes

1 tablespoon avocado oil

3 tablespoons almond flour

½ teaspoon baking powder

Pinch of kosher salt

1 large egg white

1. Pour the avocado oil in a 4-inch microwave-safe
   ramekin or bowl with a flat bottom and swirl to
   coat the bottom and sides.

2. Add the almond flour, baking powder, salt, and
   egg white. Stir well to combine. Tap the container
   on the counter a few times to remove air bubbles.

3. Microwave on high for 90 seconds. Let cool for
   1 minute and slice in half lengthwise to use as
   bread. Toast in a skillet or the toaster for an even
   better texture!

Makes 1 bread; 1 per serving | Per serving: Calories: 315, Fat: 28g, Total CARBS: 5g, Fiber: 2g, Protein: 11g

GARLICKY CRISPY CROUTONS

Making a crunchy crouton is no small feat when it comes to keto. These are perfectly crispy and garlicky and go perfectly on any salad or as just a snack.

Prep Time: 5 minutes | Cook Time: 20 minutes | Total Time: 25 minutes

½ cup almond flour

2 teaspoons garlic powder

1 teaspoon baking powder

½ teaspoon kosher salt

4 large eggs

¼ cup avocado oil

1. Preheat the oven to 400°F and spray a 12 × 8–inch baking sheet well with cooking spray.

2. Combine all the ingredients in a large mixing bowl and whisk well.

3. Pour the batter onto the prepared baking sheet. Bake for 10 minutes or until a toothpick inserted in the center comes out clean.

4. Let cool completely on the baking sheet. Once cooled, cut into 1-inch pieces.

5. Spread the cut croutons on a larger baking sheet. Spray them with cooking spray and toss to coat. Spread them back out in a single layer, leaving space in between the croutons if possible (this helps them get dry and crunchy). Place back into the oven for 10 minutes more or until golden brown and crispy.

Makes 8 servings | Per serving: Calories: 142, Fat: 13g, Total CARBS: 2g, Fiber: 1g, Protein: 5g

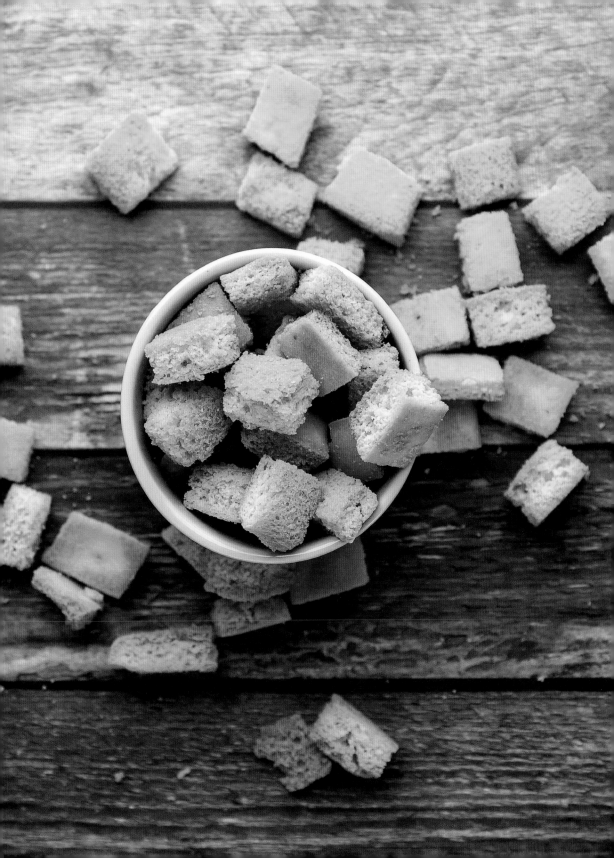

HOMEMADE RANCH DRESSING

Most ranch dressings you find in the stores are filled with questionable ingredients, so I like to make my own. You can never go wrong with homemade! This is the perfect dressing for a salad or used as a delicious dip for veggie sticks.

Prep Time: 10 minutes | Total Time: 10 minutes

1 cup mayonnaise

½ cup half-and-half

¼ cup fat-free Greek yogurt

2 tablespoons lemon juice

1 tablespoon dried parsley

1 teaspoon dried dill

1 teaspoon dried chives

1 teaspoon garlic powder

1 teaspoon onion powder

¼ teaspoon kosher salt

¼ teaspoon pepper

Makes 2 cups; 16 servings (2 tablespoons per serving) | Per serving: Calories: 107, Fat: 11g, Total CARBS: 2g, Fiber: 0g, Protein: 1g

Combine all ingredients in a medium-sized mixing bowl and whisk to combine. Transfer to a 32-ounce jar with a tight-fitting lid and store in the refrigerator for up to 2 weeks.

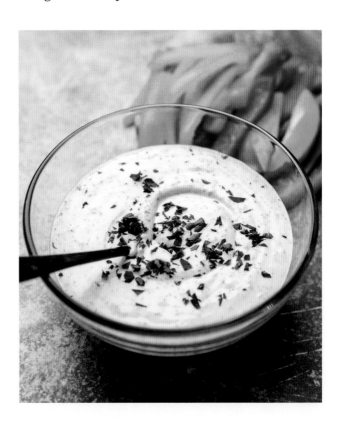

LIGHTENED-UP BLUE CHEESE DRESSING

When I am looking to cut calories but need to keep all the flavor in my salmon salads, I use this dressing recipe. Yes, only 33 calories per serving! It's also great as a dip or sandwich spread.

Prep Time: 10 minutes | Total Time: 10 minutes

7 ounces plain unsweetened fat-free Greek yogurt

⅓ cup half-and-half

1 tablespoon white wine vinegar

½ teaspoon garlic powder

½ teaspoon kosher salt

½ teaspoon pepper

2 ounces crumbled blue cheese

Makes 1¼ cups; 10 servings (2 tablespoons per serving) | Per serving: Calories: 33, Fat: 2g, Total CARBS: 1g, Fiber: 0g, Protein: 3g

Combine all ingredients, except the blue cheese, in a medium-sized mixing bowl and whisk to combine. Fold in the blue cheese. Transfer to a 32-ounce jar with a tight-fitting lid and store in the refrigerator for up to 2 weeks.

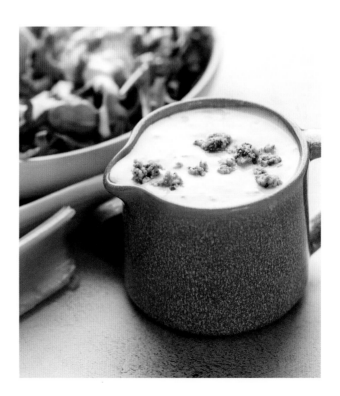

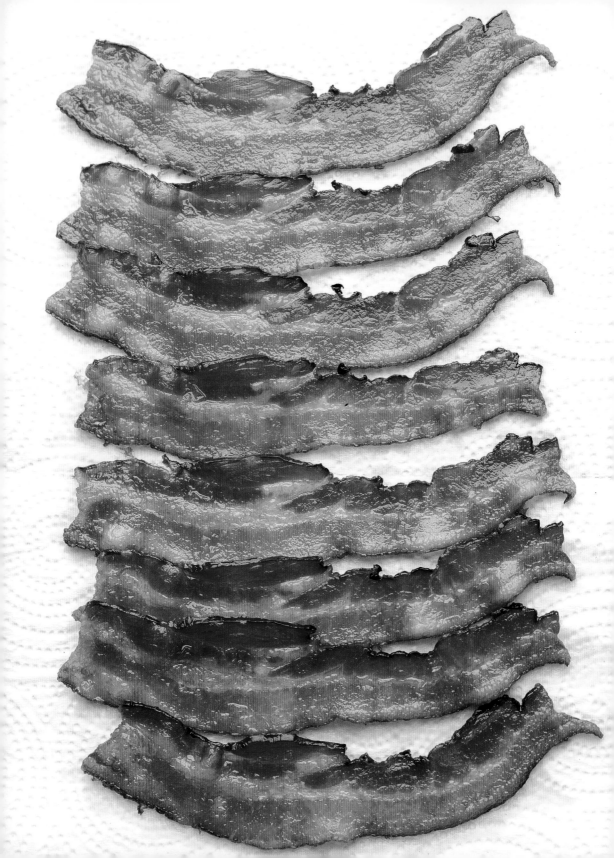

OVEN-COOKED BACON

I never ever cook bacon on the stovetop since perfecting this oven-cooked bacon. I cook a big pan each week for meal prep—you can do the same, so you always have cooked bacon on hand for recipes like Cobb Salad Meal Prep (page 111), Gruyère Mashed Cauliflower (page 228), or Jalapeño Popper Chicken Casserole (page 165), or for a quick bite at breakfast. It's the best!

Prep Time: 5 minutes | Cook Time: 20 minutes | Total Time: 25 minutes

8 slices thick bacon

1. Line a baking sheet with parchment paper or aluminum foil. Lay the bacon on the sheet tray in a single layer.

2. Place the tray in a cold oven. Set the oven to 400°F and cook for 20 minutes or until crisp to your liking. (We do not want to preheat the oven as that can lead to unevenly cooked bacon.)

3. Remove the bacon from the pan to a plate lined with paper towels to drain the grease.

Note: If you want to keep your oven clean, you can top the bacon with another sheet of parchment paper. This will keep the hot bacon grease from splattering in your oven, but it may increase the cooking time.

Makes 4 servings; 2 slices per serving | Per serving: Calories: 160, Fat: 14g, Total CARBS: 0g, Fiber: 0g, Protein: 10g

STRAWBERRY JAM

One of my favorite foods is toast with lots of butter and strawberry jam. With this keto-friendly strawberry jam and my microwave bread, it's no longer off limits!

Prep Time: 5 minutes | Cook Time: 10 minutes | Total Time: 15 minutes

10 ounces whole strawberries, chopped (about 9 large strawberries)

½ cup water

⅓ cup granulated sweetener

1 tablespoon lemon juice

1 teaspoon xanthan gum

Makes 1⅓ cups; 2 tablespoons per serving | Per serving: Calories: 11, Fat: 0g, Total CARBS: 3g, Fiber: 1g, Protein: 0g

1. Combine all of the ingredients in a small saucepan over high heat and bring to a boil. Reduce heat to medium and cook for 5 minutes, stirring frequently.

2. Remove from the heat and set aside to cool completely.

3. Pour into jelly jars with tight-fitting lids and store in the refrigerator for up to 2 weeks.

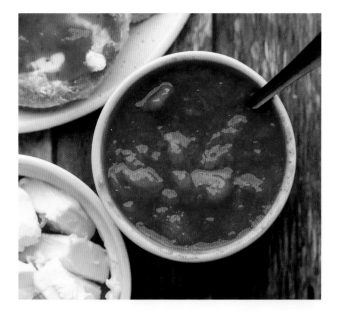

TERIYAKI SAUCE

I love a good stir-fry, and this sauce, some meat, and vegetables are all you need! If you have a gluten allergy, you can use tamari or coconut aminos in place of the soy sauce.

Prep Time: 5 minutes | Cook Time: 5 minutes | Total Time: 10 minutes

3 tablespoons brown sugar sweetener

1 garlic clove, minced

1 teaspoon grated ginger

¼ teaspoon xanthan gum

½ cup water

¼ cup soy sauce

Makes approximately ¾ cup; 3 tablespoons per serving | Per serving: Calories: 14, Fat: 0g, Total CARBS: 2g, Fiber: 1g, Protein: 2g

In a small saucepan over medium heat, combine all ingredients and bring to a boil. Let simmer until the xanthan gum completely dissolves. Remove from the heat and set aside. Use it as a sauce for your favorite stir-fry. To store: cool completely and store in an airtight container in the refrigerator for up to 2 weeks.

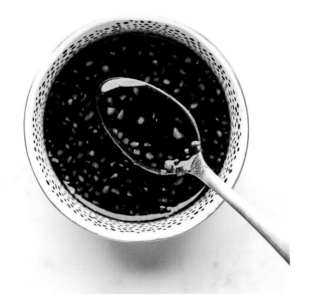

METRIC CONVERSIONS

US Standard	UK
¼ teaspoon	¼ teaspoon (scant)
½ teaspoon	½ teaspoon (scant)
¾ teaspoon	½ teaspoon (rounded)
1 teaspoon	¾ teaspoon (slightly rounded)
1 tablespoon	2½ teaspoons
¼ cup	¼ cup minus 1 dessert spoon
⅓ cup	¼ cup plus 1 teaspoon
½ cup	⅓ cup plus 2 dessert spoons
⅔ cup	½ cup plus 1 tablespoon
¾ cup	½ cup plus 2 tablespoons
1 cup	¾ cup and 2 dessert spoons

ACKNOWLEDGMENTS

First and foremost to my readers, I am so lucky that I get to do what I do and it is all because of you. Thank you so much for supporting me over the years and loving my easy approach to keto cooking. I will always deliver a logical, never complicated or dogmatic approach to keto.

I want to thank my mother, Julianne, who has been there for me and has been pivotal in the development and making of the recipes in this cookbook as well as on my blog. Without her, this cookbook would not have been imaginable.

A big thank-you to my amazing social media manager and assistant writer, Tami, who is not only a perfect sister-in-law but a great taste tester! She has kept my social media running when I couldn't bear to look at it anymore.

I want to give a giant thank-you to my editor, Claire. She gives the most amazing feedback, has been extremely patient, and has made my first real cookbook seem much easier than I thought it was ever going to be.

To the entire BenBella team, you gave me a beautiful cookbook I can be proud of. Thank you for giving me this opportunity.

And last but not least to Stacey Glick, my dear agent, thank you for finding a great home for me and my beloved cookbook. Your tireless efforts on my behalf did not go unnoticed or unappreciated.

INDEX

ABOUT THE AUTHOR

Jennifer Banz is a blogger and lover of keto. She shares her experience with her loyal followers on her Facebook page, Low Carb Recipes with Jennifer; on her YouTube channel under the same name; and on her popular recipe blog, JenniferBanz.com. Jennifer lives with her amazing husband, Matt, and two wonderful children, Hayden and Audrey, in Arkansas.